To Our Mothers

Contents

Preface

The third edition of *Nuclear Medicine Technology Examination Review* has been completely revised to reflect the many changes that have occurred in nuclear medicine instrumentation, radiopharmaceuticals, and clinical practice.

Although the book has been extensively changed to reflect the many changes in the field of nuclear medicine, the basic aim of the volume remains the same. It is intended to assist nuclear medicine technologists in assessing their knowledge of the field and to serve as an aid in reviewing further professional exams. We have again tried to emphasize the areas that are most important to the working technologist.

Nuclear medicine is not an exact science, and because of this, conflicts as to technique may occur. We have tried to select the most widely used clinical techniques in accepted practice. Furthermore, as nuclear medicine is a fast changing field, parts of this book may become obsolete quickly.

We wish to express our thanks to Janette Brown, Janet Cox, Geraldine Snider, and Deborah Williams for their help in the preparation of the manuscript.

1. BASIC PHYSICS

DIRECTIONS: Each of the questions or incomplete statements below is followed by a list of suggested answers or completions. Select the **one** that is **BEST** in each case.

---

1. Nuclear medicine is the application of ____________ materials to the diagnosis and treatment of disease.
A. nuclear
B. atomic
C. radioactive
D. chemical
REF: 18-p. 1

2. Mass and inertia are properties of
A. light
B. x-rays
C. matter
D. neutrinos
REF: 1-p. 3

3. A combination of atoms having a definite form and structure is called a(n)
   A. atomic structure
   B. mixture
   C. molecule
   D. nucleus
   REF: 19–p. 23

4. A ____________ is the smallest division of a substance having the physical properties of that substance.
   A. mixture
   B. molecule
   C. nucleus
   D. isotope
   REF: 11–p. 20

5. The smallest division of matter which can be achieved by chemical means is called a(n)
   A. mixture
   B. nucleus
   C. molecule
   D. element
   REF: 19–p. 20

6. The orderly arrangement of the chemical properties of the elements is called the
   A. mird phamplets
   B. periodic table
   C. nuclear structure tables
   D. Roentgen table
   REF: 11–p. 14

7. The electron volt (e.V.) is a unit of
   A. voltage
   B. power
   C. energy
   D. electric charge
   REF: 1–p. 24

8. Energy that has the ability to do work by reason of position is called ____________ energy.
   A. kinetic
   B. potential
   C. thermal
   D. electromagnetic
   REF: 19-p. 2

9. The Angstrom is a unit of
   A. energy
   B. length
   C. mass
   D. charge
   REF: 1-p. 29

10. The law of electrical force is known as
   A. Bohr's law
   B. Coulomb's law
   C. Einstein's law
   D. Planck's law
   REF: 1-p. 5

11. Like electrical charges ____________ each other.
   A. attract
   B. repel
   REF: 1-p. 5

12. The term used to describe all forms of electromagnetic radiation is
   A. phonon
   B. photon
   C. pion
   D. parton
   REF: 1-p. 28

13. Electromagnetic radiation is a form of ____________ radiation.
   A. wave
   B. particulate
   C. characteristic
   D. atomic
   REF: 1-p. 25

14. For electromagnetic radiation, the ____________ is the distance from a point on the wave to the same point on the subsequent wave.

A. velocity
B. frequency
C. wavelength
D. angstrom
REF: 1-p. 26

15. The three variables: wavelength (λ), frequency (ν), and velocity (c), are related by

A. $c\lambda = \nu$
B. $c\nu = \lambda$
C. $\lambda\nu = c$
D. $c = \lambda/\nu$
REF: 1-p. 26

16. Ultraviolet light has a ____________ wavelength than gamma rays.

A. longer
B. shorter
REF: 1-p. 27

17. Visible light has a ____________ frequency than x-rays.

A. higher
B. lower
REF: 1-p. 27

18. Increasing the frequency of a gamma ray ____________ its wavelength.

A. increases
B. decreases
REF: 1-p. 26

19. The speed at which a wave moves through a medium is called its

A. velocity
B. frequency
C. wavelength
D. angstrom
REF: 1-p. 26

20. The number of waves which pass a point in a unit of time is called
A. velocity
B. frequency
C. wavelength
D. angstrom
REF: 1-p. 26

21. The speed of all gamma rays is approximately
A. 3.0×10^{10} cm/sec
B. 3.0×10^{2} cm/scc
C. 6.0×10^{15} cm/sec
D. 6.0×10^{20} cm/sec
REF: 1-p. 25

22. The equation which relates the energy (E) of electro-magnetic radiation to its frequency (ν) is
A. $E = h\nu$
B. $E = h/\nu$
C. $E = \nu/h$
D. $E = h\nu^2$
REF: 1-p. 29

23. In the previous question, h is termed
A. Einstein's constant
B. Planck's constant
C. the photon factor
D. the nuclear constant
REF: 1-p. 29

24. An equation which relates the energy (E) of a photon to its wavelength (λ) is
A. $E = h\lambda$
B. $E = c\lambda$
C. $E = hc\lambda$
D. $E = hc/\lambda$
REF: 1-p. 29

25. If one measures E in electron volts and λ in angstroms
A. $E = 12400/\lambda$
B. $E = 12400\lambda$
C. $E = 12.4/\lambda$
D. $E = 12.4\,\lambda$
REF: 1-p. 29

THE FOLLOWING QUESTIONS REQUIRE THE USE OF THESE CONSTANTS:

$h = 4.13 \times 10^{-18}$keV-sec $hc = 12.4 \times 10^{-8}$keV-cm

26. What is the energy of a 5.6×10^{19}Hz gamma ray?
A. 73 keV
B. 186 keV
C. 135 keV
D. 231 keV
REF: 1-p. 29

27. What is the energy of a gamma ray with a 21×10^{-9}cm wavelength?
A. 5.9 keV
B. 6.4 keV
C. 59 keV
D. 64 keV
REF: 3-p. 29

28. What is the energy of an x-ray with a wavelength of 13×10^{-9}cm?
A. 13.2 keV
B. 1.75 keV
C. 30.8 keV
D. 9.5 keV
REF: 1-p. 29

29. What is the wavelength of a 175 keV gamma ray?
A. 7×10^{-10}cm
B. 7×10^{-11}cm
C. 7×10^{-12}cm
D. 7×10^{-13}cm
REF: 1-p. 29

30. If the wavelength of an x-ray is 5.7×10^{-13}cm, what is its frequency?
A. 4.2×10^{20}Hz
B. 8.6×10^{18}Hz
C. 5.3×10^{21}Hz
D. 17×10^{22}Hz
REF: 1-p. 28

31. If the wavelength of green light is 5 x 10^{-5}cm, what is its frequency?
A. 1.67 x 10^{15}Hz
B. 3.4 x 10^{14}Hz
C. 15 x 10^{10}Hz
D. 6 x 10^{14}Hz
REF: 1-p. 28

32. If the frequency of an x-ray is 2.5 x 10^{20}Hz, what is its wavelength?
A. 7.5 x 10^{10}cm
B. 8.3 x 10^{-10}cm
C. 1.2 x 10^{-10}cm
D. 1.2 x 10^{10}cm
REF: 1-p. 78

33. What is the wavelength of an 8 keV x-ray?
A. 12.4 x 10^{-8}cm
B. 15.4 x 10^{-9}cm
C. 12.4 x 10^{-9}cm
D. 16.2 x 10^{-9}cm
REF: 1-p. 29

34. What is the frequency of a 35 keV gamma ray?
A. 8.5 x 10^{18}Hz
B. 145 x 10^{19}Hz
C. 105 x 10^{18}Hz
D. 10.2 x 10^{20}Hz
REF: 1-p. 29

35. What is the energy of a 1.36 x 10^{20}Hz gamma ray?
A. 329 keV
B. 562 keV
C. 573 keV
D. 757 keV
REF: 1-p. 29

36. What is the frequency of a 100 keV x-ray?
A. 4.5 x 10^{20}Hz
B. 24 x 10^{18}Hz
C. 20 x 10^{19}Hz
D. 41 x 10^{18}Hz
REF: 1-p. 29

37. If the frequency of a gamma ray is 12×10^{18} Hertz, what is its wavelength?
A. 4×10^{6}cm
B. 2.5×10^{-9}cm
C. 3.6×10^{-4}cm
D. 4.6×10^{-5}cm
REF: 1-p. 28

38. The difference between light waves and x-rays is due to their
A. energies
B. sources
C. speeds
D. masses
REF: 1-p. 19

39. The only difference between x-rays and gamma rays is their
A. energy
B. source
C. speed
D. mass
E. none of the above
REF: 1-p. 20

40. Alpha particles differ from gamma rays in that alpha particles
A. have greater velocity
B. are more energetic
C. have lower frequencies
D. possess mass
REF: 1-p. 36

41. Gamma rays differ from x-rays in that they have different
A. masses
B. charges
C. velocities
D. none of the above
REF: 1-p. 49

42. Compared to electrons, gamma rays have a charge of
A. 1
B. 0
C. -1
D. -2
REF: 1-p. 49

43. Removal of an electron of a neutral atom is called
A. excitation
B. ionization
C. pairing
D. bonding
REF: 19-p. 27

44. In the excitation of an atom
A. an electron is raised to a higher energy level
B. an electron is freed from the atom
C. a positron is created
D. the nucleus is given more energy
REF: 1-p. 23

45. Radiation that has sufficient energy to remove electrons from atoms is called
A. λ-rays
B. x-rays
C. ionizing radiation
D. photon
REF: 19-p. 4

46. The atomic shells represent different
A. energy levels
B. binding energies
C. neither A nor B
D. both A and B
REF: 1-p. 21

47. The number of electrons in a shell is indicated by
A. n
B. 2n
C. n^2
D. $2n^2$
REF: 1-p. 7

48. The atomic shell which is closest to the nucleus is the
A. J-shell
B. K-shell
C. L-shell
D. M-shell
REF: 1-p. 21

49. Helium normally has its ____________-shell full.
A. K
B. L
C. M
D. N
REF: 1-p. 10

50. Atoms that show little chemical activity have their outer shell
A. filled
B. empty
C. short one electron
D. with an extra electron
REF: 11-p. 14

51. The maximum number of electrons in the L-shell is
A. 2
B. 4
C. 6
D. 8
REF: 1-p. 7

52. A transition from the L-shell to the K-shell will produce radiation of greater energy than will a transition from the M-shell to the L-shell in the same atom.
A. Always true
B. Sometimes true
C. Always false
REF: 1-p. 20

53. A certain atom has a K-shell binding energy of 70 keV and an L-shell binding energy of 8 keV. If an electron makes a transition from the L to the K-shell, the radiation emitted will have ____________ energy.
A. 78 keV
B. 70 keV
C. 62 keV
D. 8 keV
REF: 1-p. 20

54. The binding energy of a K-shell electron in iodine is approximately
A. 3 keV
B. 30 keV
C. 300 keV
D. 3 MeV
REF: 18-p. 278

55. The relationship $E = mc^2$ was originally proposed by
A. Curie
B. Einstein
C. Planck
D. Roentgen
REF: 1-p. 30

2. NUCLEAR PHYSICS

DIRECTIONS: Each of the questions or incomplete statements below is followed by a list of suggested answers or completions. Select the **one** that is **BEST** in each case.

---

56. Radioactive decay is a series of ____________ events.
A. equally spaced
B. random
C. coordinated
D. predictable
REF: 1-p. 35

57. The energy which would be required to remove a particle from the nucleus is the
A. mass energy
B. gamma energy
C. transition energy
D. binding energy
REF: 12-p. 15

58. The difference between the mass of the nucleus and the sum of the masses of the individual particles is called
A. atomic mass
B. nuclear mass
C. mass defect
D. binding capacity
REF: 1-p. 21

59. The decay of ^{32}P to ^{32}S is an example of
A. isometric decay
B. isotonic decay
C. isobaric decay
D. isotopic decay
REF: 1-p. 39

60. An alpha-particle will have ____________ two neutrons and two protons.
A. more mass than
B. the same mass as
C. less mass than
REF: 1-p. 21

61. Which of the following is NOT true of isotopes?
A. They have the same Z number
B. They have the same A number
C. They have different A numbers
D. They have the same chemical properties
REF: 1-p. 17

62. Although isotopes have the same number of protons,
A. they have different nuclear charges
B. they have different Z numbers
C. they have different number of electrons
D. they have different atomic weights
REF: 12-p. 10

63. The proton is more than ____________ times more massive than the electron.
A. 10
B. 100
C. 1000
D. 10,000
REF: 1-p. 8

64. Most stable nuclei have more ____________ than ____________.
A. electrons; protons
B. electrons; neutrons
C. protons; neutrons
D. neutrons; protons
REF: 12-p. 14

65. Which of the following affects the rate of radioactive decay?
A. Temperature
B. Pressure
C. Chemical composition
D. None of the above
REF: 1-p. 35

66. A nucleus which has more energy than it has in the ground state is said to be in a(n) ____________ state.
A. positive
B. negative
C. excited
D. stable
REF: 1-p. 49

67. Nuclei in excited states can return to the ground state by the emission of a(n)
A. β-particle
B. α-particle
C. γ-ray
D. neutrino
REF: 12-p. 21

68. In gamma ray emission, the mass number (A) changes by
A. -1
B. 0
C. +1
D. +2
REF: 1-p. 49

69. In gamma ray emission, the atomic number (Z) changes by
A. -1
B. 0
C. +1
D. +2
REF: 1-p. 49

70. In gamma ray emission, the neutron (A-Z) changes by
A. -1
B. 0
C. +1
D. +2
REF: 1-p. 49

71. A lower case "m" following the mass number (A) indicates that the nucleus is
A. stable
B. a positron emitter
C. in a metastable state (isomer)
D. fissionable
REF: 1-p. 49

72. An excited state of a nucleus which has a relatively long half-life is called an ____________ state.
A. isotopic
B. isotonic
C. isometric
D. isobaric
REF: 12-p. 22

73. Isometric states return to the ground state by emission of a(n)
A. alpha particle
B. beta ray
C. positron
D. gamma ray
REF: 1-p. 49

74. If an excited state returns to the ground state but does NOT emit a gamma ray, it will emit
A. a positron
B. internal conversion electron
C. a β^--particle
D. A and B
REF: 12-p. 23

75. If an excited nucleus returns to the ground state by internal conversion
A. an electron is emitted
B. an electron is captured
C. a gamma ray is emitted
D. the atomic number (Z) increases
REF: 1-p. 53

76. Following internal conversion, the atom usually emits
A. an alpha particle
B. an auger electron
C. a positron-electron pair
D. a characteristic x-ray
E. either B or D
F. A and D
REF: 1-p. 53

77. The β^--particle is the same as a(n)
A. electron
B. proton
C. neutron
D. positron
REF: 1-p. 38

78. The mass of the β^--particle is ____________ the mass of a proton.
A. much lighter than
B. the same as
C. slightly heavier than
D. much heavier than
REF: 12-p. 19

79. In β^- decay, the beta particle usually carries off less than the energy available (E_{max}, transition energy) because

A. the nucleus retains part of the energy
B. part of the energy is transferred to the atomic electrons
C. a neutron carries off part of the energy
D. a neutrino carries off part of the energy
REF: 1-p. 40

80. In addition to the β^- particle, a ____________ is always emitted in β^--decay.

A. neutron
B. neutrino
C. gamma ray
D. positron
REF: 12-p. 19

81. In the decay ${}^{32}_{15}P \rightarrow {}^{A}_{Z}S + \beta^- + \bar{\nu}$

A. A = 33; Z = 16
B. A = 32; Z = 14
C. A = 33; Z = 14
D. A = 32; Z = 16
REF: 1-p. 39

82. In β^--decay, the number of neutrons in the nucleus

A. decreases by two
B. decreases by one
C. remains the same
D. increases by one
REF: 12-p. 19

83. In β^--decay, the number of protons in the nucleus

A. decreases by two
B. decreases by one
C. remains the same
D. increases by one
REF: 1-p. 39

84. In β^--decay, the atomic number (Z) always changes by
A. -2
B. -1
C. 0
D. +1
REF: 12-p. 19

85. In β^--decay, the atomic mass number (A) always changes by
A. -2
B. -1
C. 0
D. +1
REF: 1-p. 39

86. In β^--decay, the total number of particles in the nucleus
A. decreases by four
B. decreases by two
C. remains the same
D. increases by one
REF: 1-p. 39

87. In β^--emission
A. the β^- preexists in the nucleus
B. the β^- is created at the moment of emission
C. the β^- comes from the atomic shells
D. the β^- is one of the atomic electrons
REF: 1-p. 39

88. In β^--decay, an average beta particle carries off approximately ____________ of the energy.
A. 5%
B. 15%
C. 33%
D. 95%
REF: 1-p. 41

89. In β^--decay, the average β^--energy is one-third of the available energy. This means
A. every β -particle has the same energy
B. every neutrino has the same energy
C. the β^- particles can have any energy from zero to the maximum but average one-third of the maximum
D. A and B
E. the β^- particles can have any energy
REF: 1-p. 40

90. The positron is similar to the electron in that it has the same
A. mass
B. charge
C. A and B
D. neither A nor B
REF: 1-p. 44

91. The positron is different from the electron in that it has a different
A. mass
B. charge
C. A and B
D. neither A nor B
REF: 1-p. 44

92. In positron decay, in addition to the positron a(n) ____________ is also emitted.
A. electron
B. neutrino
C. proton
D. alpha particle
REF: 1-p. 44

93. Positron emission is unlike β^--decay because
A. the positron is monoenergetic
B. the neutrino carries off all the energy
C. the positron always has more than half of the energy
D. none of the above
REF: 12-p. 25

94. In positron decay, the atomic number (Z) changes by
A. -2
B. -1
C. 0
D. +1
REF: 1-p. 45

95. In positron decay, the number of neutrons
A. increases by one
B. stays the same
C. decreases by one
D. decreases by two
REF: 12-p. 25

96. In positron decay, the mass number (A) changes by
A. -2
B. -1
C. 0
D. +1
REF: 1-p. 45

97. In positron decay, one of the ____________ in the nucleus is changes to a(n)
A. neutrons; proton
B. neutrons; electron
C. protons; neutron
D. protons; electron
REF: 1-p. 44

98. In the decay ${}^{A}_{Z}N \rightarrow {}^{12}_{6}C + \beta^{+} + \nu$
A. A = 13; Z = 7
B. A = 13; Z = 6
C. A = 12; Z = 7
D. A = 12; Z = 6
REF: 1-p. 47

99. In electron capture, the electron is usually captured from
A. the K-shell
B. the L-shell
C. one of the outer shells
D. the free electron population
REF: 1-p. 47

100. In electron capture, the neutron number (A-Z) changes by
A. +1
B. 0
C. -1
D. -2
REF: 1-p. 47

101. In electron capture, the mass number (A) changes by
A. +1
B. 0
C. -1
D. -2
REF: 1-p. 47

102. In electron capture, the atomic number (Z) changes by
A. +1
B. 0
C. -1
D. -2
REF: 1-p. 47

103. Electron capture is followed at once by the emission of
A. a neutron
B. a characteristic x-ray
C. auger electron
D. a positron
E. A and D
F. either B or c
REF: 1-p. 47

104. In the decay $^{68}_{32}Ge + e^- \rightarrow {}^{A}_{Z}Ga + \nu$
A. A = 67; Z = 33
B. A = 68; Z = 33
C. A = 67; Z = 31
D. A = 68; Z = 31
REF: 1-p. 65

105. An α-particle is a ____________ nucleus.
A. hydrogen-3
B. helium-3
C. helium-4
D. helium-5
REF: 12-p. 126

106. When a nucleus undergoes α-decay, its atomic number (Z) changes by
A. 0
B. -1
C. -2
D. -4
REF: 12-p. 27

107. When a nucleus undergoes α-decay, its mass number (A) changes by
A. 0
B. -1
C. -2
D. -4
REF: 12-p. 27

108. In the reaction $^{226}_{88}Ra \rightarrow ^{A}_{Z}Rn + \alpha$
A. A = 224; Z = 86
B. A = 222; Z = 86
C. A = 224; Z = 84
D. A = 222; Z = 84
REF: 12-p. 27

109. The Becquerel (Bq) is
A. 1 dps
B. 1 dpm
C. 1 dph
D. 1 dpd
REF: 12-p. 33

110. A curie is equal to ____________ nuclei decaying per second.
A. 3.7×10^{10}
B. 3.7×10^{8}
C. 3.7×10^{7}
D. 3.7×10^{5}
REF: 12-p. 33

111. Six millicuries are equal to ___________ MBq (mega Becquereles)
A. 222
B. 162
C. 22
D. 16
REF: 12-p. 33

112. The physical half-life (T_p) is related to the decay constant (λ) by
A. $\lambda T_p = 1$
B. $\lambda / T_p = 1$
C. $\lambda T_p = 0.693$
D. $\lambda / T_p = -0.693$
REF:

113. The decay constant (λ) is
A. the fraction of nuclei which decay per unit time
B. the rate of radioactive decay
C. the rate at which radiation dose is delivered
D. A and B
E. A and C
REF: 12-p. 32

114. The activity of a sample (A) with a decay constant (λ) at time (t), with an original activity (A_o) is given by
A. $A_o = Ae^{-\lambda t}$
B. $A = A_o e^{\lambda t}$
C. $A = A_o e^{\lambda / t}$
D. $A = A_o e^{-\lambda t}$
REF: 12-p. 34

115. If one plots the activity of a sample versus time on semi-logarithmic paper, one obtains a
A. parabola
B. hyperbola
C. straight line
D. none of the above
REF: 12-p. 36

QUESTIONS 116-130: THESE QUESTIONS REQUIRE THE USE OF AN EXPONENTIAL TABLE OR CALCULATOR.

116. P-32 has a half-life of 14.3 days. A sample has an original activity of 200 mCi. How much will be left after 3 days?
A. 173 mCi
B. 175 mCi
C. 179 mCi
D. 184 mCi
REF: 12-p. 34

117. O-15 has a decay constant of 0.335 min^{-1}. How much of a 15 mCi sample of ^{15}O will remain after 5 minutes?
A. 1.5 mCi
B. 2.8 mCi
C. 4.2 mCi
D. 5.6 mCi
REF: 1-p. 59

118. Hg-197 has a decay constant of 0.0107 hr^{-1}. If a sample of Hg-197 has an original activity of 300 μCi, what will its activity be after 1 week?
A. 73 μCi
B. 62 μCi
C. 50 μCi
D. 41 μCi
REF: 1-p. 59

119. A sealed source of $^{137}_{55}Cs$ has an original activity of 15 mCi. What will its activity be after 1 year? ($T_{1/2}$ = 30 yr)
A. 14.7 mCi
B. 14.4 mCi
C. 14.4 mCi
D. 13.8 mCi
REF: 1-p. 59

120. The effective half-life for a certain radiopharmaceutical is 73 days. If 50 μCi is injected into a patient on March 15, what will the activity in the patient be on June 1?
A. 18 μCi
B. 22 μCi
C. 24 μCi
D. 26 μCi
REF: 1-p. 59

121. At 3:00 p.m., a sample of ^{99m}Tc has an activity of 270 mCi. What was its activity at 8:00 a.m.?
A. 423 mCi
B. 475 mCi
C. 534 mCi
D. 606 mCi
REF: 1-p. 59

122. A Co-57 marker source has an original activity of 700 μCi. What will its activity be after 200 days? ($T_{1/2}$ = 270 da)
A. 215 μCi
B. 419 μCi
C. 530 μCi
D. 570 μCi
REF: 1-p. 59

123. Fe-59 has a decay constant $\lambda = 0.015$ da^{-1}. What percentage of an Fe-59 source will remain after 74 days?
A. 21%
B. 28%
C. 33%
D. 45%
REF: 1-p. 59

124. I-130 has a half-life of 12.4 hours. A sample of I-130 assays at 30 μCi at noon today. What was its activity at 3:00 p.m. yesterday?
A. 107 μCi
B. 97 μCi
C. 86 μCi
D. 74 μCi
REF: 1-p. 59

125. C-11 has a half-life of 20.3 minutes. What percentage of a sample of C-11 will remain after 1 hour?
A. 16.3%
B. 15.4%
C. 12.9%
D. 10.2%
REF: 1-p. 59

126. Sr-85 has a half-life of 64 days. A sample of Sr-85 assays at 200 μCi today. What was its activity 100 days ago?
A. 450 μCi
B. 520 μCi
C. 538 μCi
D. 589 μCi
REF: 1-p. 59

127. In-113m has a decay constant of 0.0069 min^{-1}. What will be the activity of a 20-mCi sample after 24 hours?
A. 0.96 μCi
B. 9.6 μCi
C. 96 μCi
D. 960 μCi
REF: 1-p. 59

128. F-18 has a decay constant of 0.0063 min^{-1}. What percentage of a sample will be left after 2 hours?
A. 35%
B. 38%
C. 47%
D. 52%
REF: 1-p. 59

129. I-125 has a half-life of 60 days. If a sample of I-125 has an activity of 2 mCi today, what will its activity be in 3 weeks?
A. 1.57 mCi
B. 1.73 mCi
C. 1.82 mCi
D. 1.85 mCi
REF: 1-p. 59

130. I-123 has a half-life of 13 hours. A sample of the material has an activity of 5.6 mCi at noon today. What was its activity at noon yesterday?
A. 10 mCi
B. 15 mCi
C. 20 mCi
D. 25 mCi
REF: 1-p. 59

QUESTIONS 131-133: REFER TO FIG. 2-1.

131. Which transition of Xe-127 has the largest internal conversion coefficient.
A. Gamma -1
B. Gamma -2
C. Gamma -3
D. Gamma -4
REF: 2 pam 10-p. 82

132. In the decay of Xe-127, which γ-ray is emitted most frequently?
A. Gamma -1
B. Gamma -3
C. Gamma -4
D. Gamma -5
REF: 2 pam 10-p. 82

133. In the decay of Xe-127 which characteristic x-ray is emitted most frequently?
A. K alpha -1
B. K alpha -2
C. K beta -1
D. K beta -2
REF: 2 pam 10-p. 82

XENON-127
ELECTRON CAPTURE DECAY

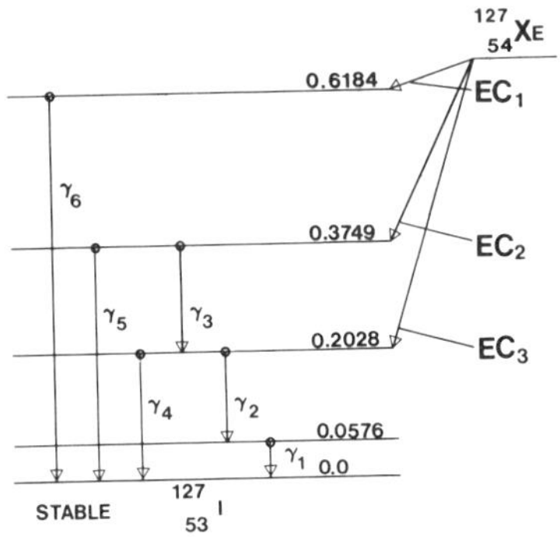

INPUT DATA

54 XENON 127 HALF LIFE = 36.4 DAYS

DECAY MODE- ELECTRON CAPTURE

TRANSITION	MEAN NUMBER/ DISINTE- GRATION	TRAN- SITION ENERGY (MEV)	OTHER NUCLEAR DATA
ELECT CAPT 1	0.0001	0.0460	ALLOWED
ELECT CAPT 2	0.4800	0.2890	ALLOWED
ELECT CAPT 3	0.5200	0.4610	ALLOWED
GAMMA 1	0.0620	0.0576	M1, AK= 2.94 K/L= 6.80 DEL= 4.70
GAMMA 2	0.0609	0.1452	E2, AK= 0.344 K/L= 3.60 DEL= 4.90
GAMMA 3	0.2970	0.1721	M1, AK= 0.158 K/L= 7.60 DEL= 4.80
GAMMA 4	0.7550	0.2028	M1, AK= 0.0975 K/L= 6.50 DEL= 5.50
GAMMA 5	0.1830	0.3749	E2, AK= 0.0148 K/L= 5.40 L/M= 8.41
GAMMA 6	0.0001	0.6184	

REF.- NUCLEAR DATA B8, 107 (1972).

OUTPUT DATA

54 XENON 127 HALF LIFE = 36.4 DAYS

DECAY MODE- ELECTRON CAPTURE

RADIATION	MEAN NUMBER/ DISINTE- GRATION n_i	MEAN ENERGY/ PAR- TICLE $\bar{E}_i$ (MeV)	EQUI- LIBRIUM DOSE CONSTANT Δ_i (g-rad/ µCi-h)
GAMMA 1	0.0137	0.0576	0.0016
K INT CON ELECT	0.0403	0.0244	0.0021
L INT CON ELECT	0.0059	0.0527	0.0006
M INT CON ELECT	0.0019	0.0567	0.0002
GAMMA 2	0.0413	0.1452	0.0128
K INT CON ELECT	0.0142	0.1120	0.0033
L INT CON ELECT	0.0039	0.1404	0.0011
M INT CON ELECT	0.0013	0.1443	0.0004
GAMMA 3	0.2504	0.1721	0.0918
K INT CON ELECT	0.0395	0.1389	0.0117
L INT CON ELECT	0.0052	0.1672	0.0018
M INT CON ELECT	0.0017	0.1712	0.0006
GAMMA 4	0.6756	0.2028	0.2918
K INT CON ELECT	0.0658	0.1696	0.0238
L INT CON ELECT	0.0101	0.1980	0.0042
M INT CON ELECT	0.0033	0.2019	0.0014
GAMMA 5	0.1797	0.3749	0.1435
K INT CON ELECT	0.0026	0.3417	0.0019
L INT CON ELECT	0.0004	0.3701	0.0003
GAMMA 6	0.0001	0.6184	0.0001
K ALPHA-1 X-RAY	0.4795	0.0286	0.0292
K ALPHA-2 X-RAY	0.2467	0.0283	0.0148
K BETA-1 X-RAY	0.1309	0.0322	0.0090
K BETA-2 X-RAY	0.0273	0.0331	0.0019
L X-RAYS	0.1419	0.0039	0.0011
KLL AUGER ELECT	0.0842	0.0235	0.0042
KLX AUGER ELECT	0.0361	0.0274	0.0021
KXY AUGER ELECT	0.0059	0.0314	0.0003
LMM AUGER ELECT	0.9413	0.0030	0.0061
MXY AUGER ELECT	2.2374	0.0008	0.0041

FIGURE 2-1. Xenon-127 electron capture decay scheme. (Reproduced with permission from L. T. Dillman and F. C. Von der Lage: Radionuclide Decay Schemes and Nuclear Parameters for Use in Radiation-Dose Estimation. *MIRD* pamphlet 10, p. 82, published by the Society of Nuclear Medicine, 1975.)

TECHNETIUM-99M
ISOMERIC LEVEL DECAY

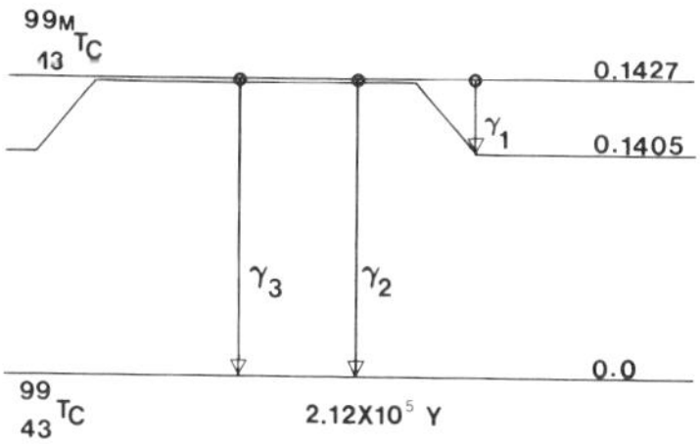

INPUT DATA

43 TECHNETIUM 99M HALF LIFE = 6.03 HOURS

DECAY MODE- ISOMERIC LEVEL

TRANSITION	MEAN NUMBER/ DISINTE- GRATION	TRAN- SITION ENERGY (MEV)	OTHER NUCLEAR DATA
GAMMA 1	0.9860	0.0021	E3
GAMMA 2	0.9860	0.1405	M1, AK= 0.104 K/L= 7.70
GAMMA 3	0.0140	0.1426	M4, AK=23.0 AL(T) = 9.21

REF.- LEDERER, C.M. ET AL, TABLE OF ISOTOPES, 6TH ED.
LEGRAND, J. ET AL, INT. J. APPL. RAD. AND ISOTOPES 21, 139 (1970).

OUTPUT DATA

43 TECHNETIUM 99M HALF LIFE = 6.03 HOURS

DECAY MODE- ISOMERIC LEVEL

RADIATION	MEAN NUMBER/ DISINTE- GRATION n_i	MEAN ENERGY/ PAR- TICLE $\bar{E}_i$ (MeV)	EQUI- LIBRIUM DOSE CONSTANT Δ_i (g-rad/ μCi-h)
GAMMA 1	0.0000	0.0021	0.0000
M INT CON ELECT	0.9860	0.0016	0.0035
GAMMA 2	0.8787	0.1405	0.2630
K INT CON ELECT	0.0913	0.1194	0.0232
L INT CON ELECT	0.0118	0.1377	0.0034
M INT CON ELECT	0.0039	0.1400	0.0011
GAMMA 3	0.0003	0.1426	0.0001
K INT CON ELECT	0.0088	0.1215	0.0022
L INT CON ELECT	0.0035	0.1398	0.0010
M INT CON ELECT	0.0011	0.1422	0.0003
K ALPHA-1 X-RAY	0.0441	0.0183	0.0017
K ALPHA-2 X-RAY	0.0221	0.0182	0.0008
K BETA-1 X-RAY	0.0105	0.0206	0.0004
KLL AUGER ELECT	0.0152	0.0154	0.0005
KLX AUGER ELECT	0.0055	0.0178	0.0002
LMM AUGER ELECT	0.1093	0.0019	0.0004
MXY AUGER ELECT	1.2359	0.0004	0.0011

FIGURE 2-2. Technetium-99m isomeric level decay scheme. (Reproduced with permission from L. T. Dillman and F. C. Von der Lage: Radionuclide Decay Schemes and Nuclear Parameters for Use in Radiation-Dose Estimation. *MIRD* pamphlet 10, p. 62, published by the Society of Nuclear Medicine, 1975.)

QUESTIONS 134-137: REFER TO FIG. 2-2.

134. The K-shell internal conversion coefficient for the gamma -2 transision is

A. 0.1405
B. 0.1194
C. 0.0913
D. 0.104
REF: 2 pam 10-p. 62

135. What is the most frequently emitted photon from Tc-99m?

A. Gamma -1
B. Gamma -2
C. Gamme -3
D. K Alpha -1 x-ray
REF: 2 pam 10-p. 62

136. In the decay of Tc-99m, which of these photons is emitted most frequently?
A. Gamma -1
B. Gamma -3
C. K Alpha -1 x-ray
D. K Alpha -2 x-ray
REF: 2 pam 10-p. 62

137. The daughter product Tc-99 is
A. stable
B. radioactive with a short half-life
C. radioactive with a medium half-life
D. radioactive with a long half-life
REF: 2 pam 10-p. 62

QUESTIONS 138-140: REFER TO FIG. 2-3.

138. The maximum energy that a β^--particle from the decay of P-32 can have is
A. 1.7100 MeV
B. 1.4799 MeV
C. 1.000 MeV
D. 0.6948 MeV
REF: 2 pam 10-p. 20

139. What is the average energy of a β^--particle from P-32 decay?
A. 1.7100 MeV
B. 1.4799 MeV
C. 1.000 MeV
D. 0.6948 MeV
REF: 2 pam 10-p. 20

140. What is the average energy of a neutrino from the decay of P-32?
A. 1.7100 MeV
B. 1.4799 MeV
C. 1.0152 MeV
D. 0.6648 MeV
REF: 2 pam 10-p. 20

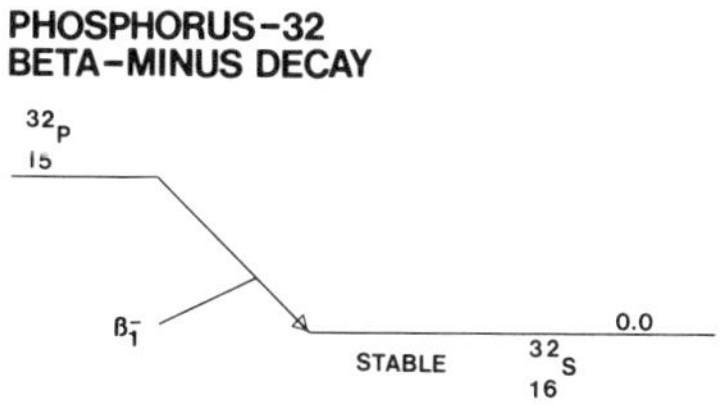

INPUT DATA

15 PHOSPHORUS 32 HALF LIFE = 14.3 DAYS

DECAY MODE- BETA MINUS

TRANSITION	MEAN NUMBER/ DISINTE- GRATION	TRAN- SITION ENERGY (MEV)	OTHER NUCLEAR DATA
BETA MINUS 1	1.0000	1.7100*	ALLOWED

*ENDPOINT ENERGY

REF.- ENDT, P.M. AND VAN DER LEUN, C., NUCL. PHYS. A105, 261 (1967).

OUTPUT DATA

15 PHOSPHORUS 32 HALF LIFE = 14.3 DAYS

DECAY MODE- BETA MINUS

RADIATION	MEAN NUMBER/ DISINTE- GRATION n_i	MEAN ENERGY/ PAR- TICLE $\bar{E}_i$ (MeV)	EQUI- LIBRIUM DOSE CONSTANT Δ_i (g-rad/ μCi-h)
BETA MINUS 1	1.0000	0.6948	1.4799

FIGURE 2-3. Phosphorus-32 beta-minus decay scheme. (Reproduced with permission from L. T. Dillman and F. C. Von der Lage: Radionuclide Decay Schemes and Nuclear Parameters for Use in Radiation-Dose Estimation. *MIRD* pamphlet 10, p. 20, published by the Society of Nuclear Medicine, 1975.)

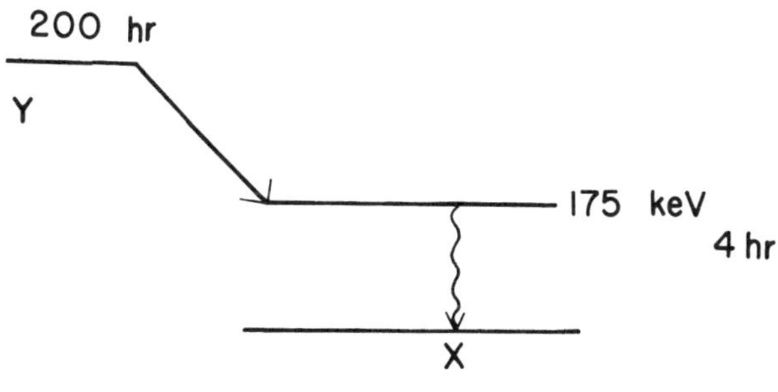

FIGURE 2-4. Decay scheme.

QUESTIONS 141-148: REFER TO THE DECAY SCHEME SHOWN IN FIG. 2-4.

141. This scheme is an example of ____________ decay.
A. beta minus
B. beta plus
C. positron
D. electron capture
REF: 1-p. 61

142. This is an example of a decay.
A. pure
B. mixed
REF: 1-p. 61

143. The decay constant for the 175 keV state is
A. 0.69 hr^{-1}
B. 0.17 hr^{-1}
C. 0.015 hr^{-1}
D. 0.0016 hr^{-1}
REF: 12-p. 36

144. The decay scheme shown would probably be suitable for a radionuclide generator.
A. True
B. False
REF: 12-p. 132

145. The state of X at 175 keV has a half-life of 4 hours. It is an example of an ____________ state.
A. isobaric
B. isotopic
C. isotonic
D. isomeric
REF: 1-p. 48

146. One begins with 400 mCi of Y. How much will be left after 600 hours?
A. 200 mCi
B. 100 mCi
C. 50 mCi
D. 25 mCi
REF: 1-p. 59

147. Nucleus X has ____________ neutron(s) than nucleus Y.
A. 1 more
B. 2 morc
C. 1 less
D. 2 less
REF: 1-p. 39

148. Nucleus X has ____________ proton(s) than nucleus Y.
A. 1 more
B. 2 more
C. 1 less
D. 2 less
REF: 1-p. 39

DIRECTIONS: Each group of questions below consists of a list of lettered headings followed by a list of numbered words or statements. For **each** numbered word or statement, select the **one** lettered heading that is most closely associated with it. Each lettered heading may be selected once, more than once, or not at all.

QUESTIONS 149-151:

A. $^{12}_{6}C$ $^{14}_{6}C$

B. $^{15}_{7}N$ $^{16}_{8}O$

C. $^{133}_{56}Ba$ $^{133}_{55}Cs$

149. isotope

150. isobar

151. isotone

REF: 12-p. 10

QUESTIONS 152-159: MATCH THE FOLLOWING NUCLIDES WITH THEIR PRINCIPAL MODE OF DECAY.

A. Alpha decay
B. Beta-minus decay
C. Positron emission
D. Electron capture

152. Co-57

153. In-111

154. I-125

155. I-131

156. Ga-67

157. Mo-99

158. P-32

159. Xe-133

REF: 2 pam 10

3. INTERACTION OF RADIATION WITH MATTER

DIRECTIONS: Each of the questions or incomplete statements below is followed by a list of suggested answers or completions. Select the **one** that is **BEST** in each case.

---

160. A charged particle moving through air loses approximately ____________ e.V. for every ion pair it produces.
A. 2
B. 20
C. 34
D. 50
REF: 12-p. 81

161. The rate at which a charged particle deposits energy along its path is termed
A. the ionization rate
B. linear energy transfer
C. energy loss factor
D. track rate constant
REF: 12-p. 143

162. If an electron and an alpha particle both have the same energy, which will have the greater LET?
A. Electron
B. Alpha particle
REF: 12-p. 143

163. The number of ion pairs per unit of track length is called
A. excitation frequency
B. specific ionization
C. RBE
D. mean free path
REF: 1-p. 38

164. A source of radiation of x-rays produces a dose rate of 50 mR/hr at 20 cm. What will the rate be at 45 cm?
A. 9.9 mR/hr
B. 12.4 mR/hr
C. 14.5 mR/hr
D. 16.8 mR/hr
REF: 1-p. 95

165. A counter 18 cm from a source of Co-60 records 72,000 cpm. The source is moved to a new distance and 44,100 cpm is recorded. What is the new distance?
A. 21 cm
B. 22 cm
C. 23 cm
D. 24 cm
REF: 1-p. 95

166. A counter, counting a sample of ^{99m}Tc, records 28,600 cpm. The source is moved from 14 cm from the counter to 8 cm from the counter. How many counts will be recorded in a minute?
A. 87,000
B. 87,260
C. 87,590
D. 87,870
REF: 1-p. 95

167. It takes 1.2 minutes to record 51,200 counts from a source of ^{131}I which is 15 cm from a detector. How long will it take to count the same number of counts if the source is moved to 58 cm?
A. 16 minutes
B. 18 minutes
C. 22 minutes
D. 24 minutes
REF: 1-p. 95

168. A therapeutic dose of ^{131}I is held in a pair of tongs 15 cm from a technologist's ring badge. The ring badge is receiving 300 mRem/hr. If shorter tongs are used and the distance is reduced to 8 cm, what will the dose rate be?

A. 1147 mRem/hr
B. 1055 mRem/hr
C. 987 mRem/hr
D. 887 mRem/hr
REF: 1-p. 95

169. A radionuclide generator stored 3 meters from a counter produces a background of 34,000 cpm. What will the background be if the generator is moved to 17 meters? (Assume there is no shielding between the generator and the counter.)

A. 106 cpm
B. 212 cpm
C. 1059 cpm
D. 2024 cpm
REF: 1-p. 95

170. Annihilation is a reaction between

A. x-rays and γ-rays
B. electrons and protons
C. protons and neutrons
D. electrons and positrons
REF: 12-p. 25

171. In annihilation, the energy released is

A. 511 keV
B. 1022 keV
C. 2048 keV
D. variable
REF: 12-p. 25

172. When a positron interacts with matter it

A. seldom annihilates
B. has a very high LET
C. sometimes produces Bremsstrahlung
D. binds to a neutron
REF: 12-p. 25

173. The range of a 1 MeV electron in water is approximately
A. 0.50 mm
B. 5 mm
C. 5 cm
D. 5 meters
REF: 12-p. 150

174. The process whereby charged particles give up part (or all) of their energy in the form of electromagnetic radiation is called
A. acceleration
B. deceleration
C. Bremsstrahlung production
D. gamma production
REF: 12-p. 138

175. The range of a 1 MeV alpha particle in water is approximately
A. 0.01 mm
B. 1 mm
C. 1 cm
D. 1 meter
REF: 12-p. 146

176. Materials with a high Z are ____________ producers of Bremsstrahlung than materials with a low Z.
A. better
B. poorer
REF: 12-p. 138

177. Alpha particles can usually be stopped by
A. a sheet of paper
B. an inch of wood
C. a foot of concrete
D. all of the above
REF: 1-p. 97

178. If an alpha particle loses an average of 34 e.V. when it creates an ion pair in air, how many ion pairs will a 680 keV alpha particle create coming to rest?
A. 20
B. 200
C. 2000
D. 20,000
REF: 1-p. 37

179. In the photoelectric process, a photoelectron is ejected from the atom. The electron
A. may have an energy less than that of the incoming photon
B. has an energy equal to that of the incoming photon
C. has an energy equal to that of the incoming photon plus the binding energy of the electron
D. has an energy equal to that of the photon minus the binding energy of the electron
REF: 12-p. 153

180. In the photoelectric process, the incoming photon
A. is completely absorbed
B. scatters with no change of energy
C. scatters with a loss of energy
D. scatters with an increase of energy
REF: 12-p. 153

181. Following a photoelectric event, an atom is most likely to emit
A. an β^--particle
B. a neutron
C. a characteristic x-ray or Auger electron
D. a α-particle from the nucleus
REF: 1-p. 51

182. The probability of a photoelectric interaction ________ with increasing Z number.
A. increases
B. decreases
REF: 12-p. 162

183. The probability of a photoelectric interaction ________ with the energy of the photon.
A. increases
B. decreases
REF: 12-p. 161

184. If the incoming photon's energy exceeds the K-shell binding energy of the atom, the photoelectric interaction will probably be with an electron from the
A. K-shell
B. L-shell
C. It depends on the Z of the atom
D. It depends on the A of the atom
REF: 12-p. 153

185. In Compton scattering, the incoming photon
A. is completely absorbed
B. scatters with no loss of energy
C. scatters with a loss of energy
D. scatters with an increase of energy
REF: 12-p. 154

186. In Compton scattering, the energy of the emitted electron
A. is equal to the energy of the incoming photon
B. is equal to half of the energy of the incoming photon
C. is equal to one-third of the energy of the incoming photon
D. none of the above
REF: 1-p. 50

187. The probability of Compton scattering ____________ with the energy of the incoming photon.
A. increases
B. decreases
C. remains the same
REF: 12-p. 162

188. In Compton scattering, the scattered photon will have the least energy if it is scattered at
A. 45 degrees
B. 90 degrees
C. 135 degrees
D. 180 degrees
REF: 12-p. 155

189. In Compton scattering, high energy photons lose ____________ fraction of the energy than (as) low energy photon if they are scattered at the same angle.
A. a greater
B. a lesser
C. the same
REF: 12-p. 155

190. A minimum of ____________ MeV is required for pair production
A. 0.51
B. 1.02
C. 5.1
D. 10.2
REF: 12-p. 157

191. In pair production, the particles which are created
A. share all of the photon's energy equally
B. share all of the photon's energy
C. share an amount of energy less than the photon's energy
REF: 1-p. 52

192. The probability that a photon will undergo pair production ____________ from 1 MeV to 10 MeV.
A. increases
B. decreases
REF: 12-p. 163

193. The probability of pair ____________ production with increasing Z.
A. increases
B. decreases
REF: 12-p. 162

194. Pair production is always followed by
A. the photoelectric effect
B. Compton scatter
C. annihilation
D. electron capture
REF: 1-p. 52

195. The relationship between the intensity of radiation and the distance from the source is
A. $I_1d_1 = I_2d_2$
B. $I_1d_2^2 = I_2d_1^2$
C. $I_1d_1^2 = I_2d_2^2$
D. $I_1d_2^2 = I_2d_1^2$
REF: 1-p. 94

196. The HVL for a certain material is 23.1 cm. What is its linear attenuation coefficient?
A. 33 cm^{-1}
B. 3.3 cm^{-1}
C. 0.3 cm^{-1}
D. 0.03 cm^{-1}
REF: 12-p. 164

197. How many half-value layers are required to reduce a beam of radiation from 200 mR/hr to 12.5 mR/hr?
A. 2
B. 3
C. 4
D. 5
REF: 1-p. 100

198. A certain material has a linear attenuation coefficient of 0.139 cm^{-1} for 100 keV gamma rays. What percentage of the beam of 100 keV gamma rays will penetrate 1.2 cm of this material?
A. 75%
B. 80%
C. 85%
D. 90%
REF: 1-p. 99

199. The HVL for annihilation radiation in lead is approximately 3.85 mm. What fraction of a beam of positrons will penetrate 2.3 cm of lead?
A. 0.10
B. 0.16
C. 0.010
D. 0.016
REF: 1-p. 99

200. Tissue has a linear attenuation coefficient of approximately 0.45 cm^{-1} for the 27 keV x-ray of ^{125}I. What percentage of these x-rays will pass through 2 cm of tissue?
A. 54%
B. 41%
C. 37%
D. 28%
REF: 1-p. 99

201. HVL for annihilation radiation in tissue is 7.7 cm. What percentage of a beam of 511 keV x-rays will penetrate 15 cm of tissue?
A. 37%
B. 34%
C. 31%
D. 26%
REF: 1-p. 99

202. The half-value layer for a certain material is 3.4 cm. How much of this material is required to reduce a beam of radiation to 25% of its original intensity?
A. 1.7 cm
B. 3.4 cm
C. 6.8 cm
D. 10.2 cm
REF: 1-p. 100

203. The relationship between the linear attenuation coefficient (μ) and the half-value layer (HVL) is given by
A. $HVL/\mu = 0.693$
B. $HVL = 0.693/\mu$
C. $HVL = 0.693\mu$
D. $HVL\mu^2 = 0.693$
REF: 12-p. 164

204. The linear attenuation coefficient ____________ with decreasing density.
A. increases
B. decreases
REF: 12-p. 161

205. In general, the linear attenuation coefficient _________ with increasing Z.
A. increases
B. decreases
REF: 12-p. 162

206. In general, the linear attenuation coefficient _________ with energy from 1 keV to 1 MeV.
A. increases
B. decreases
REF: 18-p. 125

207. The linear attenuation coefficient depends on the
A. energy of the photon only
B. attenuating material only
C. both energy and attenuating material
D. the photon energy, attenuating material, and the speed of the photon
REF: 12-p. 162

208. The most probable interaction of a 50 keV gamma ray in tissue is
A. photoelectric effect
B. Compton scattering
C. pair production
REF: 12-p. 162

209. A 5 keV gamma ray is most likely to interact with water by
A. photoelectric effect
B. Compton scatter
C. pair production
REF: 12-p. 162

210. The attenuation of radiation by x cm of matter with a linear attenuation coefficient of μ is described by

A. $I - I_o x^2$

B. $I = I_o^2 e^{-\mu x}$

C. $I = I_o e^{\mu x}$

D. $I = I_o e^{-\mu x}$

REF: 12-p. 163

211. Lead has a linear attenuation coefficient of approximately 25 cm^{-1} for the 140 keV gamma ray of ^{99m}Tc. What fraction of these gamma rays will pass through 0.8 mm of lead?

x: 25 x .08 = 2 e^{-2} = .135

A. 0.128

B. 0.130

C. 0.135

D. 0.142

REF: 1-p. 99

4. COUNTING INSTRUMENTATION

DIRECTIONS: Each of the questions or incomplete statements below is followed by a list of suggested answers or completions. Select the **one** that is **BEST** in each case.

---

212. Which of the following is not a gas detector?

A. "Cutie pie"
B. Gamma camera
C. GM counter
D. Dose calibrator
REF: 1-p. 131

213. Dose calibrators are examples of

A. ionization chambers
B. NaI (Tl) scintillation spectrometers
C. Geiger counters
D. none of the above
REF: 12-p. 259

214. Dose calibrators are superior to NaI (Tl) well counters for assaying radioactive material because
A. they can count high activity better than an NaI (Tl) scintillation spectrometer
B. they do not need to be calibrated
C. they are more sensitive to radiation than well counters
D. A and B
E. A and C
REF: 12-p. 259

215. One of the advantages of the "cutie pie" as a survey meter is that
A. it responds only to contamination
B. its reading isn't strongly dependent on the energy of the gamma rays
C. it responds only to high energy radiation
D. none of the above
REF: 12-p. 50

216. The "cutie pie" is a(n) ____________ counter.
A. gas flow
B. sodium-iodide
C. Geiger-Muller
D. ionization
REF: 12-p. 52

217. If insufficient voltage is applied to the electrodes of an ionization chamber
A. the radiation will fail to ionize the gas
B. the ions created will recombine before reaching the electrodes
C. electric current will not be able to flow in the circuit
D. the ions will not properly penetrate the electrodes
REF: 12-p. 51

218. In an ionization chamber run in the saturation region, the current is directly proportional to the
A. type of radiation
B. energy of the radiation
C. voltage applied to the electrodes
D. number of ions created in the gas
REF: 1-p. 133

219. In the proportional region, the number of ions collected is increased by the
A. proportional effect
B. avalanche effect
C. Compton effect
D. photoelectric effect
REF: 1-p. 135

220. In the proportional region, the ions in the gas gain sufficient energy to
A. cause Bremsstrahlung
B. create additional ions
C. penetrate the collection electrode
D. cause Compton scatter
E. A and B
REF: 1-p. 135

221. The most common use of the proportional counter in clinical medicine is
A. dose calibration
B. low energy gamma-counting
C. positron counting
D. checking for alpha-emitting contaminants
REF: 1-p. 136

222. Many proportional detectors are
A. gas flow counters
B. "cutie pie" counters
C. dose calibrators
D. used as personal monitors
REF: 1-p. 135

223. In the Geiger region, the ions in the gas gain sufficient energy to
A. cause Bremsstrahlung
B. create additional ions
C. cause Compton scatter
D. penetrate the collection electrode
E. A and B
REF: 1-p. 136

224. The voltage below which a Geiger-Muller tube will not count is called the
A. starting potential
B. threshold
C. plateau
D. operating voltage
REF: 59-p. 10

225. A Geiger counter is restored to its normal quiescent state by a process called
A. dead time
B. quenching
C. positive ion loss
D. wall depolarization
REF: 12-p. 58

226. A Geiger-Muller tube which is reaching the end of its useful life will show
A. a lower starting potential
B. an increased slope of the plateau
C. a decreased slope of the plateau
D. a great increase in efficiency
REF: 59-p. 12

227. The correct operating voltage of Geiger-Muller tubes should be within the ____________ 25% of the plateau.
A. 1st
B. 2nd
C. 3rd
D. 4th
REF: 59-p. 12

228. The ____________ should be used for low-level surveys since it is more sensitive than the ____________.
A. Geiger-Muller; "cutie pie"
B. "cutie pie"; Geiger-Muller
C. "cutie pie"; ionization
D. "cutie pie"; gas flow
REF: 59-p. 9

229. When using a source to calibrate a survey meter, it should be
A. kept away from scattering material
B. more than 15 mCi
C. sent to NBS for calibration
D. placed in water to simulate a patient
REF: 2-p. 6

230. A material which emits light when struck by ionizing radiation is called a(n)
A. crystal detector
B. ion chamber
C. scintillator
D. photon detector
REF: 12-p. 64

231. The most commonly used scintillation material in the nuclear medicine laboratory is
A. CsI (Tl)
B. NaI (Tl)
C. zinc cadminum sulfide
D. calcium tunstate
REF: 1-p. 137

232. Material which is hygroscopic
A. readily absorbs water
B. repels water
C. is sensitive to x-rays
D. always scintillates poorly
REF: 1-p. 138

233. The amount of light emitted by an NaI (Tl) crystal depends upon the
A. diameter of the crystal
B. thickness of the crystal
C. energy of the gamma ray
D. energy absorbed in the crystal
REF: 3-p. 139

234. If it is necessary to locate the scintillator at some distance from the PM tube, a(n) ___________ is used.
A. electron pipe
B. gamma pipe
C. light pipe
D. magnesium oxide pipe
REF: 5-p. 211

235. The basic function of a photomultiplier tube is to convert ___________ into ___________.
A. gamma rays; electrical pulse
B. x-rays; photons
C. light; electrical pulse
D. none of the above
REF: 12-p. 64

236. At the photocathode of a photomultiplier tube, _______ knock ___________ loose.
A. photons; electrons
B. photons; gamma rays
C. electrons; x-rays
D. electrons; photons
REF: 12-p. 64

237. The process described in the previous question is called
A. Compton scatter
B. photoelectric effect
C. vacuum absorption
D. electron capture
REF: 12-p. 64

238. In a photomultiplier tube, the electrons interact with a series of
A. photocathodes
B. cathodes
C. anodes
D. dynodes
REF: 12-p. 65

239. The output of a photomultiplier tube is proportional to
A. the energy the gamma ray deposits in the scintillation crystal
B. the energy of the emitted gamma ray
C. neither of the above
REF: 12-p. 68

240. Changes in the high voltage level cause changes in the gain of the photomultiplier tube because it affects
A. secondary emission
B. electrons produced at photocathode
C. A and B
REF: 1-p. 140

241. The gain of a photomultiplier tube is very sensitive to
A. the energy of the gamma rays striking the scintillation crystal
B. the high voltage applied to the tube
C. A and B
D. neither A nor B
REF: 12-p. 66

242. The three functions of a preamplifier in an NaI (Tl) scintillation spectrometer are
A. energy selection, amplification, and impedance matching
B. high voltage control, amplification, and pulse shaping
C. pulse shaping, impedance matching, and amplification
D. amplification, high voltage control, and energy selection
REF: 12-p. 74

243. In an NaI (Tl) scintillation detector, the preamplifier is usually attached directly to the
A. NaI (Tl) crystal
B. photomultiplier tube
C. single-channel analyzer
D. scaler
REF: 1-p. 140

244. Another term for single-channel analyzer is
- **A.** postamplifier
- **B.** scaler
- **C.** pulse height analyzer
- **D.** ratemeter

REF: 1-p. 143

245. A scaler is designed for
- **A.** counting single pulses from a detector
- **B.** determining the maximum count rate from a radionuclide
- **C.** determining the rate at which pulses are being counted
- **D.** determining the length of time a radionuclide has been counted

REF: 3-p. 153

246. A pulse height analyzer consists of which three circuits?
- **A.** Upper level discriminator, lower level discriminator, and coincidence circuit
- **B.** Upper level discriminator, lower level discriminator, and anti-coincidence circuit
- **C.** Baseline control and coincidence and anti-coincidence circuits
- **D.** Baseline control and upper and lower level coincidence circuits

REF: 12-p. 82

247. Increasing the time constant of an analog ratemeter ____________ the fluctuations which will be observed in the output.
- **A.** increases
- **B.** decreases

REF: 1-p. 155

QUESTIONS 248-260: FOR THESE QUESTIONS, CONSIDER AN NaI (Tl) SCINTILLATION SPECTROMETER WITH A NORMAL GAIN SWITCH, WITH GAINS OF 1, 2, AND 4. IT IS EQUIPPED WITH A SINGLE CHANNEL ANALYZER WHICH HAS A BASELINE THAT ADJUSTS FROM 1 TO 1000, AND A DIFFERENTIAL WINDOW THAT ALSO ADJUSTS FROM 0 TO 1000. THE UNIT IS CALIBRATED WITH THE GAIN SET AT 2, SO THAT EACH DIVISION ON THE SCA IS EQUAL TO 1 keV.

248. A good source to use for the calibration would be
A. Cs-137
B. Ga-67
C. I-125
D. I-131
REF: 59-p. 23

249. The original calibration would be done by adjusting
A. the source position
B. the amplifier gain
C. the high voltage
D. the preamplifier gain
REF: 59-p. 26

250. The window width used on the SCA should be about ____________ for calibration.
A. 0.5%
B. 3%
C. 15%
D. 30%
REF: 59-p. 25

FOR COUNTING A SAMPLE OF ^{198}Au (412 keV PEAK) WITH A 15% WINDOW:

251. The baseline of the SCA should be set at
A. 350
B. 381
C. 412
D. 443
REF: 1-p. 143

252. The window should be set at
A. 31
B. 62
C. 93
D. 124
REF: 3-p. 143

ONE WISHES TO COUNT THE 320 keV PEAK OF ^{51}Cr WITH A 10% WINDOW:

253. The window should be set at
A. 8
B. 16
C. 32
D. 64
REF: 1-p. 143

254. The baseline of the SCA should be set at
A. 288
B. 304
C. 320
D. 336
REF: 1-p. 143

255. In counting an unknown sample, a peak is found with the baseline at 240 and the window at 36. The energy of the peak is
A. 204 keV
B. 240 keV
C. 258 keV
D. 225 keV
REF: 1-p. 142

ONE WISHES TO COUNT ^{60}Co WITH AN ACCEPTABLE ENERGY RANGE FROM 1050 TO 1400 keV:

256. The gain should be set at
A. 1
B. 2
C. 4
REF: 59-p. 41

257. The baseline should be set to
- **A.** 525
- **B.** 625
- **C.** 1050
- **D.** 1400

REF: 59-p. 41

258. The window should be set at
- **A.** 44
- **B.** 88
- **C.** 175
- **D.** 350

REF: 59-p. 41

259. With the gain set at 4, the baseline at 56, and the window at 12, a peak is found. What is the energy of the peak?
- **A.** 12 keV
- **B.** 31 keV
- **C.** 56 keV
- **D.** 62 keV

REF: 59-p. 41

260. With the gain at 1, the baseline at 785, and the window at 50, a peak is found. What is the energy of the peak?
- **A.** 785 keV
- **B.** 810 keV
- **C.** 1570 keV
- **D.** 1595 keV

REF: 59-p. 41

QUESTIONS 261-267: REFER TO FIG. 4-1.

261. The peak at "A" is called the ____________ peak.
- **A.** Compton
- **B.** differential
- **C.** photopeak
- **D.** scintillation

REF: 12-p. 195

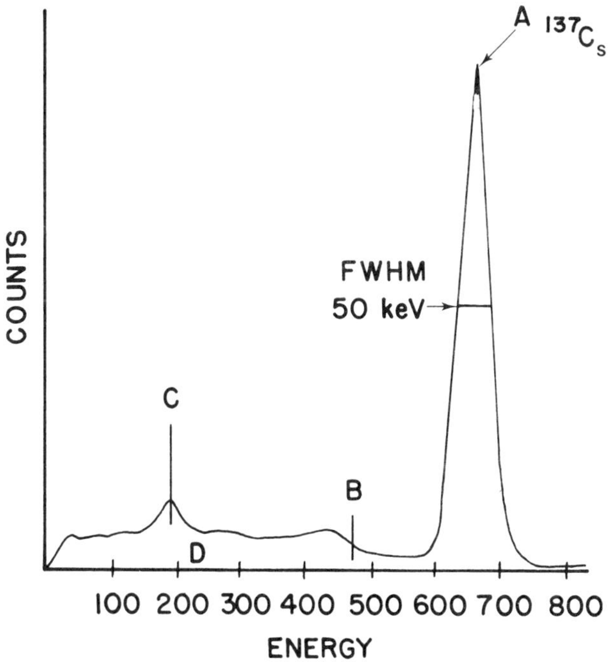

FIGURE 4-1.

262. This peak "A" is composed of gamma rays which
- **A.** interact in the crystal and deposit all their energy there
- **B.** interact only by the photoelectric effect
- **C.** interact only by the Compton scatter
- **D.** none of the above

REF: 12-p. 195

263. The resolution for peak "A" is approximately
- **A.** 2%
- **B.** 7.5%
- **C.** 15%
- **D.** 18%

REF: 12-p. 195

264. The point labeled "B" is called the
A. photoedge
B. Compton edge
C. scatter endpoint
D. backscatter peak
REF: 12-p. 185

265. The area labeled "D" is due to
A. Compton scattered radiation
B. electrical noise
C. pair production escapes
D. β^--particles
REF: 12-p. 185

266. If one were to use a smaller NaI (Tl) crystal, the ratio of area "A" to area "D" would
A. increase
B. decrease
REF: 12-p. 185

267. The small peak at "C" is called a ___________ peak.
A. photo
B. backscatter
C. Compton
D. electron
REF: 12-p. 217

268. When counting ^{125}I, a window from approximately 15 keV to 80 keV is usually used. This is done to
A. minimize scatter
B. decrease absorption of x-rays in the crystal's encapsulation
C. reject the sum peak
D. include the sum peak
REF: 12-p. 185

269. The performance of clinical counting equipment should be checked
A. each day
B. once a week
C. once a month
D. whenever trouble is suspected
REF: 5-p. 229

270. Most electronic equipment functions best if it is
A. turned off when not in use
B. turned off overnight
C. left on all the time
REF: 5-p. 228

271. The efficiency of a detector is defined as the ratio of counts/unit time to
A. crystal size
B. emission rate
C. activity in mCi
D. none of the above
REF: 12-p. 209

272. Intrinsic efficiency is defined as the ratio of total-absorption scintillations to total ____________ photons.
A. emitted
B. incident
C. absorbed
D. counted
REF: 12-p. 212

273. When one is at some distance from the crystal, its geometric efficiency is given by: (r = radius of detector; d = distance from source to crystal)
A. $\pi r^2/d^2$
B. $r^2/4\pi d^2$
C. $r^2/4d^2$
D. $4r^2/d$
REF: 12-p. 210

274. The geometric efficiency of a 5-inch diameter NaI (Tl) crystal for a source 10 inches from the crystal is
A. 16.3%
B. 6.3%
C. 16%
D. 1.6%
REF: 12-p. 210

275. The geometric efficiency of a 3-inch diameter NaI (Tl) crystal for a source 8 inches from the crystal is

A. 15%
B. 1.5%
C. 9%
D. 0.9%
REF: 12-p. 210

276. In using a well counter, a tube is not set in the well properly so that the tube is elevated 1 cm. This will ____________ the efficiency of the counter.

A. increase
B. decrease
C. leave unchanged
REF: 61-47:10

277. The efficiency of a well counter ____________ with increasing sample volume.

A. increases
B. decreases
C. remains the same
REF: 61-47:11

278. Because the efficiency of a well counter changes with sample volume, it is necessary to

A. calibrate the counter for geometric effects
B. use samples and standards which have the same volume
C. A and B
D. either A or B
REF: 61-47:11

279. In counting, the standard deviation (σ) in the number of counts (N) is

A. $\sqrt{1/2N}$
B. $1\sqrt{1/2N}$
C. $\sqrt{N}$
D. $2\sqrt{N}$
REF: 1-p. 214

280. The probability that a count will fall within one standard deviation of the true count is

A. 50%
B. 68%
C. 73%
D. 95%
REF: 1-p. 215

281. The 2σ confidence level is

A. 62%
B. 85%
C. 95%
D. 98%
REF: 1-p. 215

282. The 3σ confidence level is

A. 92%
B. 95%
C. 97%
D. 99%
REF: 1-p. 215

283. The standard deviation of 8000 counts is

A. 89
B. 93
C. 179
D. 268
REF: 3-p. 214

284. Two standard deviations of 79,000 counts is

A. 281
B. 562
C. 843
D. 1124
REF: 1-p. 214

285. The standard deviation of 54,000 counts is

A. 232
B. 274
C. 298
D. 567
REF: 1-p. 214

286. If one observes a count rate (R) for a time (t), the standard deviation of the rate (σR) is

A. $2\sqrt{Rt}$
B. $2\sqrt{R/t}$
C. $\sqrt{R/t}$
D. $\sqrt{Rt}$
REF: 12-p. 109

287. The number of counts (N) required to achieve a percent error (V) at 2 confidence level is

A. 10,000/V
B. $10{,}000/V^2$
C. 40,000/V
D. $40{,}000/V^2$
REF: 1-p. 216

288. How many counts are required to attain a 2 confidence level 5%?

A. 100
B. 400
C. 1600
D. 8000
REF: 3-p. 217

289. For the previous question, the standard deviation for the true count rate (σRt) is

A. $\sqrt{R_o/t_o + R_b/t_b}$
B. $\sqrt{R_o/t_o - R_b/t_b}$
C. $\sqrt{R_o t_o + R_b t_b}$
D. $\sqrt{R_o t_o - R_b t_b}$
REF: 12-p. 109

290. If one has an observed count rate (R_o) and a background count rate (R_b) for times t_o and t_b, the true count rate (R_t) is

A. $R_t = R_o + R_b$
B. $R_t = R_o - R_b$
C. $R_t = R_o/t_o - R_b/t_b$
D. $R_t = R_o t_o - R_b t_b$
REF: 12-p. 109

291. A sample is counted for 5 minutes and 58,000 counts are attained. A background run of 10 minutes produced 4000 counts. The true count rate is

A. 54,000 counts
B. 27,000 counts
C. 11,200 cpm
D. 10,400 cpm
REF: 12-p. 109

292. For the data in the previous question, what is the standard deviation of the true count rate?

A. 124 cpm
B. 118 cpm
C. 65 cpm
D. 49 cpm
REF: 12-p. 109

293. The count rate for a sample is 10 cpm for 20 minutes. A background rate of 5 cpm for 30 minutes is measured. What is the standard deviation of the true count rate?

A. 0.8 cpm
B. 1.1 cpm
C. 1.8 cpm
D. 2.3 cpm
REF: 12-p. 109

294. A count rate of 45 cps is observed for a 10 second time. A background of 30 cps is observed for 15 seconds. What is the true count rate?

A. 45 cps
B. 30 cps
C. 15 cps
D. 10 cps
REF: 12-p. 109

295. For the previous question, what is the standard deviation of the true count rate?

A. 2.5 cps
B. 3.0 cps
C. 3.5 cps
D. 4.0 cps
REF: 12-p. 109

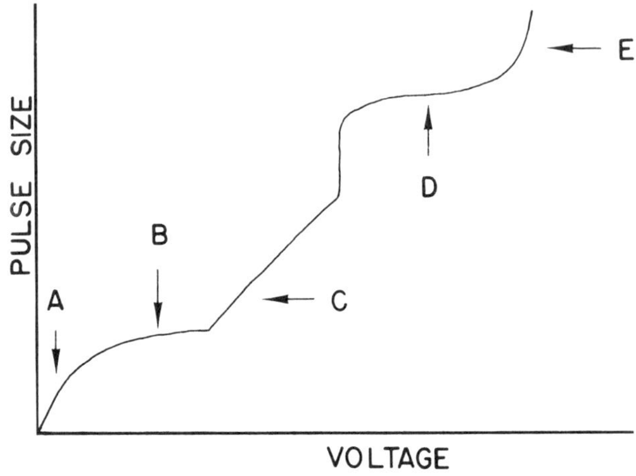

FIGURE 4-2.

DIRECTIONS: Each group of questions below consists of a list of lettered headings or a diagram with lettered components followed by a list of numbered words or statements. For **each** numbered word or statement, select the **one** lettered heading that is most closely associated with it. Each lettered heading may be selected once, more than once, or not at all.

QUESTIONS 296-306: REFER TO FIG. 4-2.

MATCH THE LETTERED DESIGNATED REGION WITH ITS PROPER NAME BELOW:

296. Continuous discharge

297. Ionization (saturation)

298. Proportional

299. Geiger–Muller (plateau)

300. Rccombination

REF: 1–p. 132

IN WHICH REGION WOULD EACH OF THE FOLLOWING INSTRUMENTS BE OPERATED? (IF NONE OF THE REGIONS ARE APPROPRIATE, ANSWER "F"):

301. Dose calibrator

302. "Cutie Pie"

303. GM survey meter

304. Pocket dosimeter

305. Well counter

306. Gamma camera

REF: 33–111:405
REF: 3–p. 133
REF: 3–p. 136
REF: 3–p. 133
REF: 3–p. 137
REF: 3–p. 165

QUESTIONS 307–315: REFER TO FIG. 4–3.

307. Amplifier

308. Preamplifier

309. Single–channel analyzer

310. Scaler

311. High voltage supply

312. Dynode

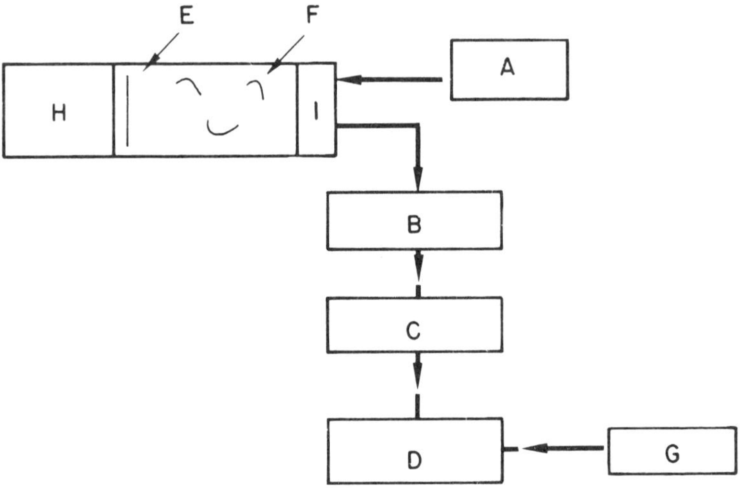

FIGURE 4–3.

313. Photocathode

314. NaI (Tl) crystal

315. Timer

REF: 1-pp. 137–156

QUESTIONS 316–322:

A. Increases intrinsic efficiency
B. Decreases intrinsic efficiency
C. Increases extrinsic or geometric efficiency
D. Decreases extrinsic or geometric efficiency
E. Leaves efficiency unchanged

316. Increasing the diameter of the crystal

317. Increasing the thickness of the crystal

318. Increasing the source strength

319. Changing the energy of a gamma ray from 200 keV to 400 keV

320. Moving the source closer to the crystal

321. Decreasing the high voltage

322. Increasing the amplifier gain

REF: 12-chap. 12

DIRECTIONS: Each of the statements below is followed by a series of options. Select either true (T) or false (F) for **each** option given.

---

323. Because there are losses due to dead time, the true count rate is always greater than the observed count rate.
REF: 59-p. 13

324. The gain of a photomultiplier tube is sensitive to magnetic fields and may change if the orientation of the detector is changed.
REF: 5-p. 216

325. In amplifiers with true gain, doubling the gain doubles the pulse height.
REF: 5-p. 141

326. The greater the time constant of a ratemeter, the greater the fluctuations it will show.
REF: 5-p. 141

5. IMAGING INSTRUMENTATION

DIRECTIONS: Each of the questions or incomplete statements below is followed by a list of suggested answers or completions. Select the **one** that is **BEST** in each case.

---

327. The detection element in a gamma camera is
- **A.** an array of cesium iodide crystals
- **B.** an array of sodium iodide crystals
- **C.** a single cesium iodide crystal
- **D.** a single sodium iodide crystal

REF: 12-p. 267

328. Modern gamma cameras usually have at least ________ photomultiplier tubes.
- **A.** 19
- **B.** 37
- **C.** 61
- **D.** 91

REF: 12-p. 267

329. The electronics in the gamma camera can determine
A. the energy of the gamma ray
B. where the gamma ray strikes the crystal
C. the dead time of the camera
D. A and B
E. all of the above
REF: 10-p. 233

330. Detector efficiency for a gamma camera is best for a ____________ mm thick crystal.
A. 6
B. 8
C. 13
REF: 12-p. 289

331. Detector efficiency ____________ with increasing gamma ray energy.
A. increases
B. decreases
C. remains the same
REF: 12-p. 289

332. A way to improve scatter rejection on a gamma camera is to use
A. a wider window
B. two windows on the same peak
C. a window offset to the high side
D. a window offset to the low side
REF: 64-p. 78

333. Because of dead time losses a gamma camera's observed count rate is less than its true count rate. This is usually not a problem except for
A. bone scans
B. first pass ventriculograms
C. Muga's
D. kidney flows
REF: 12-p. 290

334. The dead time of typical gamma camera is about
A. 10 picoseconds
B. 10 microseconds
C. 100 microseconds
D. 10 milliseconds
REF: 12-p. 290

335. The field of view of a standard gamma camers is about
A. 15 cm
B. 25 cm
C. 39 cm
D. 49 cm
REF: 5, Vol. 7, p. 305, 1977

336. The field of view of a large field of view gamma camera is about
A. 15 cm
B. 25 cm
C. 38 cm
D. 49 cm
REF: 5, Vol. 7, p. 305, 1977

337. Usually ____________ collimators have the best resolution and poorest efficiency.
A. converging
B. diverging
C. parallel hold
D. pinhole
REF: 12-p. 301

338. If a gamma camera has two parallel hole collimators with the same hole diameter and septal thickness, the ____________ collimator will have better resolution at 10 cm depth.
A. thicker
B. thinner
C. there will be no difference
REF: 12-p. 293

339. Most gamma camera imaging is done with a _________ collimator.
A. pinhole
B. parallel hole
C. diverging
D. converging
REF: 12-p. 272

340. Which gamma camera collimator will have the lower MTF?
A. High sensitivity
B. High resolution
REF: 1-p. 227

341. The high ____________ collimator for a gamma camera has a faster falloff of resolution with depth than the high ____________ collimator.
A. sensitivity; resolution
B. resolution; sensitivity
REF: 10-p. 407

342. An image of the thyroid is being done on a gamma camera equipped with a pinhole collimator. The pinhole has an aperture of 1.5 mm. The thyroid to pinhole distance is 8 cm and the pinhole to crystal distance is 16 cm. On the crystal, the thyroid is
A. reduced by a factor of two
B. magnified by a factor of two
C. magnified by a factor of three
D. not enough date are given to answer the question
REF: 12-p. 271

343. For the data of the previous question, if you move the camera closer to the thyroid, the magnification will
A. increase
B. decrease
REF: 12-p. 271

344. Intrinsic resolution refers to
A. the resolution that can be obtained under ideal circumstances (without scatter, etc.)
B. the resolution that can be obtained by the crystal alone
C. the resolution that can be obtained by the crystal and electronics
D. the resolution of the crystal, electronics, and collimator
REF: 12-p. 287

345. Which crystal size has the best intrinsic resolution?
A. 6 mm
B. 8 mm
C. 13 mm
REF: 12-p. 288

346. A gamma camera will have the best intrinsic resolution for which radionuclide?
A. Ga-67
B. I-131
C. Tc-99m
D. Tl-201
REF: 12-p. 288

347. The underlying cause of nonuniformity in the gamma camera that causes the greatest nonuniformity is
A. noninformities in the crystal
B. noninformity in PM tubes
C. nonlinearities
D. pulse pile up
REF: 12-p. 287

348. The chief advantage of a multicrystal camera is that it has ____________ than a conventional gamma camera.
A. better spatial resolution
B. better energy resolution
C. better efficiency
D. lower dead time
REF: 12-p. 315

349. Tomographic images that are obtained by SPECT imaging with a rotating gamma camera are usually reconstructed using the ____________ method.
A. unfiltered back projection
B. filtered back projection
C. ARTS method
D. linear interpolation
REF: 64-p. 97

350. A difficulty of SPECT as compared to PET is
A. back projection
B. determining the energy of the gamma rays
C. attenuation corrections
D. image projection
REF: 64-p. 100

351. The chief advantages of PET is its
A. low cost
B. short imaging time
C. ability to do physiological studies with positron-emitting radionuclides
D. its ability to do very fast studies of myocardial function
REF: 12-p. 324

352. If the modulation transfer function (MTF) of a collimator is MTFc and the MTF of the crystal is MTFx, the combined MTF is
A. MTFc + MTFx
B. MTFc x MTFx
C. MTFc/MTFx
D. MTFx/MTFc
REF: 12-p. 335

353. If collimator A has resolution that is twice as good as collimator B, the efficiency of collimator A will be ____________ that of collimator B.
A. 1/4
B. 1/2
C. 2 times
D. 4 times
REF: 12-p. 296

354. If a computer was a 16 bit word, a byte will be _______ bits.
A. 4
B. 8
C. 16
D. 32
REF: 64-p. 117

355. A 128 x 128 matrix will have ___________ pixels.
A. 4096
B. 8192
C. 16,384
D. 32,768
REF: 64-p. 119

356. The device that takes the output of a gamma camera and converts it to form useable by the computer is called a(n)
A. CPU
B. FTA
C. MMPI
D. ADC
REF: 64-p. 122

357. The part of the computer that controls the other parts is called the
A. CPU
B. FTA
C. MMPI
D. ADC
REF: 64-p. 119

6. QUALITY CONTROL

DIRECTIONS: Each of the questions or incomplete statements below is followed by a list of suggested answers or completions. Select the **one** that is **BEST** in each case.

---

358. An important principle of quality control is
A. use only Tc-99m source
B. establish a protocol and follow it exactly
C. measure uniformity daily
D. measure uniformity with collimator off
REF: 2-p. 339

359. An unsatisfactory scan which occurs between two satisfactory scans is most likely due to
A. an intermittent instrument failure
B. line voltage fluctuations
C. photomultiplier tube burnout
D. operator error
REF: 5-p. 234

360. You have just received a new well counter. The first test that should be done is
A. chi-square test
B. energy resolution
C. energy calibration
D. spatial resolution
REF: 59-p. 121

361. You are now doing an energy resolution measurement with a 10 keV window using the 662 keV energy of Cs-137

Base Line	Count
700	2500
690	4500
680	6900
670	8800
660	9900
650	9500
640	7800
630	5200
620	3500
610	2100

The full width at half maximum (FWHM) is
A. 52 keV
B. 61 keV
C. 57 keV
D. 68 keV
REF: 59-p. 140

362. In order to find the % resolution, which formula does one use?
A. $\% \text{ Resolution} = \frac{\text{FWHM}}{662}$
B. $\% \text{ Resolution} = \frac{\text{FWHM}}{662} \times 100$
C. $\% \text{ Resolution} = \text{FWHM} \times 662$
D. $\% \text{ Resolution} = (\text{FWHM} + 10)/662$
REF: 59-p. 140

363. The % Resolution is
- **A.** 9.4%
- **B.** 9.2%
- **C.** 9.0%
- **D.** 8.8%

REF: 59-p. 140

364. A good test to measure the short-term stability of the counter is
- **A.** energy resolution
- **B.** 60 cycle test count
- **C.** chi-square test
- **D.** daily test count

REF: 59-p. 128

365. The formula for finding chi-square is
- **A.** $\chi^2 = \frac{(Ni - N)^2}{N}$
- **B.** $\chi^2 = \frac{(Ni - N)}{N}$
- **C.** $\chi^2 = \frac{N}{(Ni - N)}$
- **D.** $\chi^2 = \frac{N}{(Ni - N)} \quad 2$

N = Avg. count; Ni = individual counts

REF: 59-p. 128

366. What is χ^2 for the following data?

16127	16160	16277	16212	16101
16207	16309	16314	16397	16279

- **A.** 4.6
- **B.** 4.8
- **C.** 5.0
- **D.** 5.2

REF: 59-p. 128

367. This corresponds to a χ^2 probability in the range
- **A.** greater than 95%
- **B.** 90 - 50%
- **C.** 50 - 10%
- **D.** less than 10%

REF: 59-p. 128

368. Is this within normal limits?
- **A.** Yes
- **B.** No

REF: 59-p. 128

369. The daily flood image for a gamma camera should
- **A.** have about 10^6 counts for a standard field, 2 x 10^6 counts for a wide field
- **B.** be collected at count rates of less than 20 K/sec
- **C.** A and B

REF: 50-p. 344

370. The PHA of a γ-camera should be set
- **A.** with the collimator off
- **B.** with the collimator on

REF: 10-p. 342

371. The display scope dots should be focused
- **A.** only when nonfocus is noted
- **B.** each day
- **C.** every time the intensity is changed
- **D.** focus is not available on most machines

REF: 10-p. 342

372. Co-57 disk sources have been found to have the following problems.
- **A.** High cost and limited lifetime
- **B.** Nonuniformities
- **C.** High energy contamination
- **D.** All the above

REF: 10-p. 338

373. For cameras that use Polaroid film it is important to
- **A.** clean the rollers several times each day
- **B.** clean the lenses monthly
- **C.** clean the oscilloscope screen monthly
- **D.** all of the above

REF: 10-p. 341

374. The line spread function is used to measure

A. energy resolution
B. spatial resolution
C. efficiency
D. focal depth
REF: 1-p. 208

375. Uniformity should be measured each ____________ for a gamma camera.

A. day
B. week
C. month
D. 6 months
REF: 5-p. 337

7. RADIATION BIOLOGY

DIRECTIONS: Each of the questions or incomplete statements below is followed by a list of suggested answers or completions. Select the **one** that is **BEST** in each case.

---

376. As an ionizing radiation passes through a cell
- **A.** cellular death is immediate
- **B.** damage to the cell may not occur
- **C.** it seeks out and destroys the most sensitive targets
- **D.** it preferentially reacts with the chromosomes

REF: 27-p. 23

377. Radiation-induced DNA damage may manifest itself as
- **A.** change in nitrogenous base sequence
- **B.** loss of a nitrogenous base
- **C.** break in the hydrogen bond between nitrogenous bases
- **D.** all of the above

REF: 28-p. 28

378. The most radiosensitive structures and/or molecules are found in
A. mitochondria
B. ribosomes
C. nucleus
D. nucleolus
REF: 29-p. 28

379. Which of the following cannot be killed by ionizing radiation?
A. Viruses
B. Bacteria
C. Plant cells
D. Animal cells
E. All can be killed
REF: 28-p. 35

380. In addition to its ability to kill cells, ionizing radiation can also
A. stimulate cellular growth
B. stimulate meiosis
C. inhibit mitosis
D. inhibit cell killing
REF: 28-p. 35

381. One (some of the) change(s) which result(s) when protein is irradiated is (are)
A. decreased molecular weight
B. cross-linking
C. fragmentation
D. all of the above
REF: 28-p. 22

382. The law of Bergonie and Tribondeau states in part that
A. highly specialized cells are radiosensitive
B. cells which are mitotically active are radioresistant
C. cells which are mitotically active are radiosensitive
REF: 25-p. 6

383. The law of Bergonie and Tribondeau also states that
- **A.** primitive or undifferentiated cells are radiosensitive
- **B.** primitive or undifferentiated cells are radioresistant
- **C.** degree of differentiation does not influence cellular radiosensitivity
- **D.** germ cells are unaffected by low doses (100 rads) or radiation

REF: 25-p. 6

384. Linear energy transfer (LET) is
- **A.** rate of energy deposition
- **B.** rate of ion pair formation
- **C.** rate of radical formation
- **D.** is used in describing electrolysis of water

REF: 27-p. 26

385. LET (linear energy transfer)
- **A.** is identical for all ionizing radiation
- **B.** is greater for particulate radiation
- **C.** is greater for electromagnetic radiation
- **D.** does not apply to ionizing radiation

REF: 30-p. 96

386. Although radiation-induced genetic mutations are identical to naturally occurring mutations
- **A.** the frequency of their occurrence is increased
- **B.** radiation-induced mutations are more selective
- **C.** radiation dose and direction can be controlled; radiation-induced mutations are beneficial
- **D.** naturally occurring genetic mutations cease to occur following irradiation

REF: 24-p. 16

387. The frequency of radiation-induced genetic mutations
- **A.** is invariably higher in germ cells
- **B.** increases with the age of the individual
- **C.** continues at an increased rate even after exposure
- **D.** increases linearly with the dose of radiation

REF: 24-p. 22

388. Most of the radiation-induced mutations are
A. dominant
B. spontaneous
C. harmful
D. selectively beneficial
REF: 23-p. 79

389. Radiation-induced genetic mutations
A. are reversible
B. are permanent
C. may be reversible or permanent depending on the type of cell in which mutation are produced
D. may be reversible or permanent depending on the type and energy of the radiation
REF: 23-p. 82

390. There is no threshold dose known for the induction of mutations. This means that
A. the dose which produces only one mutation is known
B. only doses above the threshold dose will result in a mutation
C. mutations may occur only as a result of a large dose of radiation
D. mutations may occur as a result of any amount of radiation
REF: 23-p. 72

391. Radiation-induced mutations are a result of
A. changes in DNA
B. changes in RNA
C. changes in the deoxyribose sugar
D. change of H_3PO_4 to H_2PO_3
REF: 28-p. 27

392. It is believed that the induction of leukemia follows irradiation by
A. 1-3 years
B. 3-5 years
C. 5-8 years
D. 8-10 years
REF: 29-p. 150

393. The earliest radiation-induced cancer is thought to be
A. squamous cell carcinoma
B. leukemia
C. bronchiogenic carcinoma
D. osteosarcoma
REF: 29-p. 150

394. Analysis of chromosomes in lymphocytes of peripheral circulation in man suggests that
A. only therapeutic external beam exposures result in an increased frequency of genetic mutations
B. certain diagnostic procedures result in an increased frequency of mutations
C. background radiation decreases the frequency of mutations
D. the rate of mutations increases linearly with age
REF: 23-p. 82

395. Within limits, mutational frequency is directly proportional to
A. type of cell involved
B. LET
C. sequence of purine bases in the DNA
D. arrangement of pyrimidine bases in the DNA
REF: 24-p. 24

396. The time interval between exposure and observable effect is called
A. dead time
B. S phase
C. metabolic period
D. latent period
REF: 24-p. 43

397. One (some) of the late effects of radiation on living systems is (are)
A. erythema
B. nonspecific life-span shortening
C. hemorrhage
D. spontaneous abortion of the fetus
REF: 27-p. 141

398. The $LD_{50/30}$ concept refers to
A. lethality in higher organisms
B. the amount of radiation required to kill 50% of the irradiated population within 30 days
C. both of the above
REF: 30–p. 209

399. The $LD_{50/30}$ for man is believed to be
A. 250 to 450 rads
B. 500 to 750 rads
C. less than 100 rads
D. more than 750 rads
REF: 25–p. 153

400. A number of factors can influence an individual's response to whole body irradiation. Among these may be
A. chronological age
B. inherent radiosensitivity
C. state of health
D. all of the above
REF: 23–p. 191

401. The factor commonly used to compare the anticipated effectiveness of two types of ionizing radiation is
A. LD_{50}
B. Compton factor
C. LET (linear energy transfer)
D. RBE (relative biological effectiveness)
REF: 30–p. 97

402. The RBE for fast neutrons for producing eye opacities is
A. 10–15 times higher than for x-rays
B. considerably lower than for x-rays
C. exactly equal to x-rays of the same keV
D. neutrons cannot be compared with photons
REF: 25–p. 295

403. The simplest and most effective means of reducing the biological response to radiation is produced by
A. administration of massive doses of normal saline
B. decreasing the amount of available oxygen, thus producing hypoxia
C. hyperbaric oxygenation
D. administration of chemicals which have a free sulfhydryl group
REF: 30-p. 81ff

404. Generally, the effects of acute vs. fractionated doses of radiation will be
A. milder with an acute dose
B. the latent period following an acute dose will be longer
C. milder following fractionated doses
D. about the same if the total dose is identical
REF: 24-p. 116

405. The earliest clinical manifestations resulting from whole-body acute exposure to a large (400 rads) dose of radiation usually is (are)
A. anxiety with tachycardia
B. nausea and vomiting
C. diarrhea
D. all of the above
REF: 23-p. 192

406. The prodromal period is
A. time periof of GI distress following acute exposure to radiation
B. apparent just before the exposure occurs
C. time period during which the patient is asymptomatic
D. apparent just before the patient dies
REF: 24-p. 135

407. Reproductive death or reproductive failure is defined as the cell's inability to
A. divide once after irradiation
B. divide twice after irradiation
C. divide repeatedly after irradiation
REF: 28-p. 35

408. An individual who dies in 3 to 10 days following an acute whole-body exposure is believed to die due to
A. hematopoietic death
B. gastrointestinal death
C. central nervous system death
D. thermal trauma
REF: 30-p. 207

409. CNS (central nervous system) death
A. occurs within a few hours following exposure
B. results from huge dose (10,000 rads or more) of whole-body acute exposure
C. is associated with lesions of the lung
D. all of the above
REF: 30-p. 207

410. A patient dying from the CNS syndrome may show an undamaged and intact gut; this is due to
A. changes in this organ may not yet be apparent
B. the gut has been protected by the alert medical team
C. CNS syndrome is secondary to gut death
D. CNS syndrome is secondary to hematopoietic death
REF: 30-p. 207

411. Radiation sickness is
A. manifested only by small laboratory animals
B. seen in man following whole-body exposure to 50 rads or more
C. a form of psychogenic reaction
D. due to skin exposure to beta radiation
REF: 24-p. 134

412. The onset, duration, and severity of the radiation sickness symptoms depend on
A. previous exposure to radiation
B. dose-rate of radiation
C. dose of radiation
D. a complicated physical-psychogenic factor
REF: 25-p. 153

413. A true GI (gastrointestinal) syndrome may result from
- **A.** fractionated exposure of the entire body
- **B.** acute exposure of the whole body
- **C.** acute exposure of the abdomen
- **D.** A and C only

REF: 24-p. 134

414. In a true GI syndrome, the patient
- **A.** experiences anorexia
- **B.** develops dehydration secondary to vomiting and diarrhea
- **C.** may show early signs of infection due to an almost total depletion of WBCs
- **D.** all of the above

REF: 24-p. 137

415. An acutely irradiated patient who survives the initial few weeks postexposure may die as a result of
- **A.** general infection
- **B.** failure of the bone marrow to repopulate the circulating blood
- **C.** hematopoietic or "bone marrow" syndrome
- **D.** all of the above

REF: 24-p. 137

416. Bone marrow and lymphoid organs
- **A.** are radioresistant
- **B.** are highly radiosensitive
- **C.** will continue to function normally following large doses of radiation
- **D.** function only when stimulated by gross hemorrhage or infection

REF: 27-p. 57

417. Even though the lymphocyte does not undergo mitosis, it is
- **A.** very radioresistant as per the law of Bergonie and Tribondeau
- **B.** very radiosensitive as an exception to the law of Bergonie and Tribondeau
- **C.** not as sensitive as a platelet
- **D.** not affected by radiation

REF: 27-p. 65

418. Changes in the hemopoietic system following irradiation may include
A. decrease in the cellular component of the circulating blood
B. appearance of reticulocytes in the circulation
C. death of many erythrocyte stem cells
D. all of the above
REF: 27-p. 72

419. The late effects of radiation
A. may never be expressed
B. may be seen months or years following exposure
C. are of little concern because they are insignificant
D. are of great concern because they inevitably kill the patient
REF: 24-p. 134

420. Ionizing radiation is a universal carcinogen because
A. like certain classes of chemicals, it will produce cancer in all species
B. like certain viruses, it will produce cancer in all species
C. unlike other carcinogens, only radiation will produce cancer in all species
D. it is used to treat cancer all over the world
REF: 24-p. 43

421. Irradiation of the embryo with small (diagnostic) amounts of radiation may result in
A. spontaneous abortion
B. multiple births
C. placenta previa
D. breech presentation
REF: 24-p. 40

422. Irradiation of the embryo between the 3rd and 6th week of pregnancy (during organogenesis) frequently results in
A. malformations
B. neonatal death
C. mental retardation
D. all of the above
REF: 24-p. 67

423. In a pregnant female, diagnostic procedures involving the use of ionizing radiation should be
A. avoided, especially during the first trimester
B. limited to the first and second trimesters
C. limited to fluoroscopic studies of the GI tract
D. used routinely to visually confirm presence of a fetus
REF: 24-p. 71

424. Radiosensitivity of the embryo changes with age so that
A. the older embryo is more sensitive than a young one
B. the younger embryo is more sensitive
C. the young embryo is only as resistant as its mother
D. the older embryo is more resistant than its mother
REF: 24-p. 66

425. Which of the following is (are) a frequently observed malformation(s) which results from irradiation of the human embryo in utero?
A. Microcephaly and mental retardation
B. Congenital dislocation of the hip
C. Congenital heart disease
D. All of the above
REF: 24-p. 66ff

426. Therapeutic doses of I^{131} used to treat carcinoma of the thyroid are
A. capable of inducing sterility in the human female
B. too low to produce somatic mutations
C. too low to produce genetic mutations
D. capable of producing the true GI syndrome
REF: 23-p. 74

427. Radionuclides of Sr, P, I, and tritium
A. cannot cross the placental barrier to the fetus
B. can cross the placental barrier and become incorporated into the fetal tissues
C. have short effective half-lives and have no effect on the fetus
D. have short biological half-lives and present no threat to the fetus
REF: 23-p. 98

428. The degree of hazard resulting from an internally deposited source of radiation depends on
A. the type and energy of the radiation emitted
B. its physical half-life
C. its biological half-life
D. all of the above
REF: 26-p. 277

429. Once inside the body, radionuclides
A. are excreted rapidly
B. become engulfed by the circulating lymphocytes as other hostile bodies
C. follow the same metabolic processes as their nonradioactive counterparts
D. become deposited and incorporated into the bony framework of the body
REF: 26-p. 279

430. Calculation of the radiation dose from internally located radionuclides is
A. very difficult
B. no more difficult than dose calculations for external beam source
C. only possible when its damage begins to be manifested
D. not possible without whole-body counter
REF: 26-p. 279

431. Internally located alpha and beta emitters are more hazardous than a gamma emitter because
A. gamma emitters are removed from the body faster than alpha and beta emitters
B. alpha and beta emitters dissipate most of their energy within a small volume of tissue within a critical organ
C. alpha and beta emitters frequently activate other elements and make them radioactive also
D. gamma emitters can be chelated and thus made stable
REF: 26-p. 276

432. In calculating the effective half-life of a radionuclide, which factor(s) must be considered?
A. Physical half-life
B. Type of emission
C. Time required for the radionuclide to reach equilibrium
D. B and C only
REF: 26-p. 477

433. The biological half-life of an element is
A. an estimate of the rate of removal of the element from the tissue
B. an estimate of the rate of decay of the element
C. a combination of A and B
D. an estimate of the expected survival of the tissue adjacent to the element
REF: 1-p. 62

434. In order to handle the radionuclide safely, the technologist must know the radionuclide's
A. chemical properties
B. physical properties
C. route of administration
D. rate of excretion
REF: 59-p. 420

435. The average annual gonadal dose of an average individual is
A. 50 mrem
B. 100 mrem
C. 150 Mrem
D. 200 mrem
REF: 30-p. 413

436. The effects of low doses of medical radiation are very difficult to determine because they may be masked by
A. effects from background radiation
B. physical injury
C. psychogenic factors
D. diurnal rhythm
REF: 24-p. 78

437. Very low doses of radiation from medical procedures are considered safe if they
- **A.** do not exceed background radiation
- **B.** are less than 5 rem per year
- **C.** do not occur during patient's pregnancy
- **D.** no amount of radiation is considered safe

REF: 59–p. 463

438. In evaluation of risk vs. benefit of medical radiation, usually
- **A.** risk clearly prevails
- **B.** benefit clearly prevails
- **C.** risk and benefit are of equal value
- **D.** need not be considered for a nonpregnant patient

REF: 24–p. 75

439. One of the risks considered in therapeutic irradiation is
- **A.** appearance of new malignancies outside the irradiated volume
- **B.** scarring of the skin outside the port area
- **C.** severe osteomalacia in the treatment area
- **D.** cosmetic effect

REF: 24–p. 75

440. One of the factors which may affect the risk of low-level medical irradiation in nuclear medicine is
- **A.** patient's diurnal rhythm
- **B.** stress
- **C.** psychogenic factors
- **D.** patient's age

REF: 24–p. 82

441. Patient's radiation dose from nuclear medicine procedures can be reduced by use of radionuclides
- **A.** which are pure gamma emitters
- **B.** with long biological half-life
- **C.** with long physical half-life
- **D.** which are equally distributed to all organs

REF: 30–p. 431

442. At diagnostic level, ultrasound has been shown to

A. damage DNA
B. be beneficial to cells undergoing mitosis
C. have very little or no effect on cells, tissues, or organs
D. produce significant hyperthermia in target organs
REF: 24-p. 155

443. Cavitation is a process by which ultrasound is

A. generated
B. propagated
C. absorbed
D. detected
REF: 24-p. 156

8. RADIATION PROTECTION

DIRECTIONS: Each of the questions or incomplete statements below is followed by a list of suggested answers or completions. Select the **one** that is **BEST** in each case.

---

444. The Roentgen is a unit which measures __________ of radiation.
A. intensity
B. quantity
REF: 1-p. 86

445. The Roentgen is NOT defined for
A. x-rays
B. gamma rays
C. beta particles
D. none of the above
REF: 1-p. 86

446. The definition of the Roentgen depends upon the ionization of
A. muscle tissue
B. water
C. air
D. dry nitrogen
REF: 1-p. 86

447. The ____________ is used to estimate a dose in rads when the exposure in Roentgens is known.
A. quality factor
B. f-factor
C. RBE
D. LET
REF: 1-p. 86

448. The rem is NOT defined for
A. gamma rays
B. beta rays
C. neutrons
D. none of the above
REF: 1-p. 87

449. The dose in rem is determined by multiplying the dose in rads by
A. the Roentgen factor
B. the relative biological effectiveness
C. the gamma constant
D. the time exposure
REF: 1-p. 87

450. For 140 keV gamma rays, the dose in rem is _________ the dose in rads.
A. less than
B. equal to
C. greater than
REF: 1-p. 87

451. For the beta particle from the decay of ^{32}P, the dose in rem is ____________ the dose in rads.
A. less than
B. equal to
C. greater than
REF: 1-p. 87

452. The dose in rem from alpha particles is ____________ the dose in rads.
A. less than
B. equal to
C. greater than
REF: 1-p. 87

453. The SI unit for absorbed dose is the
A. RAD
B. REM
C. Gray
D. Sievert
REF: 12-p. 171

454. An absorbed dose of 50 joules/kg is equal to
A. 500 REM
B. 50 RADs
C. 50 Gray
D. 500 Sievert
REF: 12-p. 171

455. The SI unit of dose equivalent is the
A. RAD
B. REM
C. Gray
D. Sievert
REF: 12-p. 347

456. A person receives an absorbed dose of 5 gray from radiation that has a quality factor of 2. What is the dose equivalence in sieverts?
A. 0.1
B. 1.0
C. 10
D. 100
REF: 12-p. 347

457. The maximum permissible prospective dose for the lens of the eye shall not exceed ____________ in any one year.
A. 1 rem
B. 5 rem
C. 15 rem
D. 25 rem
REF: 63-p. 89

458. The maximum permissible prospective dose to the red bone marrow shall not exceed ____________ in any one year.
A. 1 rem
B. 5 rem
C. 15 rem
D. 25 rem
REF: 63-p. 89

459. A pregnant nuclear medicine technologist should
A. be placed on leave as soon as it is determined that she is pregnant
B. be allowed to work until the 8th month of pregnancy
C. be transferred to a position in which she will receive no radiation
D. be carefully evaluated so that there is no danger of her receiving more thn 0.5 rem of radiation
REF: 63-p. 92

460. Pregnant nurses should cease being responsible for the routine care of patients with appreciable radioactive burdens
A. as soon as their pregnancy is discovered
B. after three months of pregnancy
C. after six months of pregnancy
D. after eight months of pregnancy
REF: 63-p. 10

461. A special duty nurse should not normally be assigned to the care of more than ____________ radioactive patients per month.
A. One
B. Two
C. Five
D. Ten
REF: 63-p. 11

462. The maximum permissible prospective dose for any one year, to the gonads, shall not exceed
A. 1 rem
B. 5 rem
C. 15 rem
D. 25 rem
REF: 63-p. 89

463. The dose limit for nonoccupationally exposed individuals does not include
A. natural radiation
B. medical radiation
C. dental radiation
D. any of the above
REF: 63-p. 95

464. The maximum permissible dose to the whole body of an individual not occupationally exposed shall not exceed ____________ rem in any one year.
A. 0.01
B. 0.05
C. 0.1
D. 0.5
REF: 63-p. 95

465. During the entire gestation period, the maximum permissible dose to the fetus from occupational exposure to the expectant mother should not exceed
A. 0.2 rem
B. 0.5 rem
C. 1 rem
D. 2 rem
REF: 63-p. 92

466. The maximum permissible dose in a single year to the hands of a radiation worker is
A. 75 mrem
B. 7.5 rem
C. 75 rem
D. 750 rem
REF: 63-p. 106

467. The prospective annual limit for whole body occupational exposure to radiation workers is
A. 1 rem per year
B. 5 rem per year
C. 15 rem per year
D. 25 rem per year
REF: 63-p. 106

468. The prospective annual limit for whole body occupational exposure to radiation workers is
A. 1 rem per year
B. 5 rem per year
C. 15 rem per year
D. 25 rem per year
REF: 63-p. 106

469. Persons under the age for full-time radiation work may be exposed to radiation for training purposes providing that the total dose for 1 year does not exceed
A. 0.1 rem
B. 0.5 rem
C. 1 rem
D. 5 rem
REF: 63-p. 99

470. The NCRP recommends that whenever possible, persons under the age of ____________ years should not be employed as full-time radiation workers.
A. 16
B. 18
C. 19
D. 21
REF: 63-p. 99

471. The radiation dose from a 10-uCi dose of ^{99m}Tc left on the skin is about
A. 1 mRad
B. 1 Rad
C. 100 Rad
D. 100,000 Rad
REF: 62-p. 86

472. In a well-run laboratory most of the dose to technologists is due to
A. injecting patients
B. radiation from patients
C. eluting generators
D. drawing up doses
REF: 62-p. 95

473. During a CBF and static brain study (20 mCi) a technologist might receive about ____________ mR to the whole body.
A. 10
B. 2
C. 1
D. 1/3
REF: 62-p. 86

474. The use of a syringe shield can reduce this dose by a factor of
A. 5
B. 70
C. 200
D. 400
REF: 62-p. 86

475. For the dose rate in the previous question, how long can one hold the syringe each day and stay under the 75 Rem/yr limit?
A. 1 second
B. 1 minute
C. 2 minutes
D. 1 hour
REF: 62-p. 86

476. The dose rate to the tip of the index finger from 20 mCi of ^{99m}Tc in 2 ml in an unshielded syringe is about
A. 20 mR/hr
B. 200 mR/hr
C. 2000 mR/hr
D. 20,000 mR/hr
REF: 62-p. 86

477. The maximum exposure rate at a specified distance from patients who have received therapeutic amounts of gamma-emitting radionuclides should be made; this measurement is usually made
A. at the body surface
B. at the foot of the patient's bed
C. at 1 meter from the patient
D. at 5 meters from the patient
REF: 63-p. 7

478. The appropriate formula for the maximum radiation accumulation of a person "n" years old is
A. 5 x n
B. (5 x n) + 18
C. (n - 18) x 5
D. (n - 5) x 18
REF: 63-p. 106

479. The maximum accumulated radiation dose to a technologist who is 28 years old is
A. 5 rem
B. 50 rem
C. 180 rem
D. 500 rem
REF: 63-p. 106

480. A technologist who is 38 years old and has never worked with radiation previously is hired by a nuclear medicine department. During her first year of work, her radiation dose should not exceed
A. 5 rem
B. 50 rem
C. 75 rem
D. 100 rem
REF: 63-p. 106

481. The radioactive precautions tag which is attached to the chart of patients who have received therapeutic amounts of gamma-emitting radionuclides, shall list all of the following EXCEPT
A. the date on which the patient may be discharged from the hospital
B. the exposure rate at 1 meter from the patient
C. the radionuclide administered
D. the activity of the radionuclide, in mCi, at the time of administration
REF: 64-p. 9

482. Patients receiving therapeutic amounts of radionuclides should normally be hospitalized until the level of activity falls below
A. 100 mCi
B. 70 mCi
C. 30 mCi
D. 10 mCi
REF: 64-p. 17

DIRECTIONS: Each of the questions or incomplete statements below is followed by a series of options. Select either (T) or false (F) for **each** option given.

---

483. A motor vehicle transporting a radioactive III package must be posted with signs indicating radioactive material.
REF: 1-p. 142

484. The surface dose of a radioactive II package must be less than 10 mR/hr.
REF: 1-p. 142

485. While eating is banned in preparation areas, it may be allowed in counting rooms.
REF: 1-p. 239

486. Nuclear medicine technologists should be equipped with finger (ring) badges.
REF: 1-p. 240

487. Nuclear medicine technologists should have their film badges changed at weekly intervals for maximum accuracy.
REF: 1-p. 230

488. It is usually permissible to dispose of the urine from Schilling's test patients in the sanitary sewer.
REF: 59-p. 151

489. It is not necessary to wear rubber gloves when handling low energy beta emitters.
REF: 59-p. 134

490. Cosmetics should not be applied in areas where radioactive materials are used.
REF: 1-p. 239

491. Protective gloves should always be worn when handling radioactive materials.
REF: 1-p. 240

492. Pipetting by mouth is allowed provided that the activity of the material is less than one microcurie per cubic centimeter.
REF: 59-p. 240

493. Patients who have been treated with therapeutic amounts of ^{131}I should have their own tableware.
REF: 6-p. 13

494. The urine from patients who have received therapeutic amounts of ^{131}I should always be collected in special containers and saved.
REF: 6-p. 13

495. Particular care must be taken in handling the vomitus of patients who have been treated with colloidal gold or phosphorus.
REF: 6-p. 14

496. In general, visitors to patients who have received therapeutic amounts of radioactive materials should stay at a distance of greater than 6 feet from the patient.
REF: 6-p. 15

9. RADIOPHARMACEUTICALS

DIRECTIONS: Each of the questions or incomplete statements below is followed by a list of suggested answers or completions. Select the **one** that is **BEST** in each case.

---

497. Fusion occurs when
A. two light nuclei coalesce to form a heavier nucleus
B. an alpha particle splits to form two deutrons
C. a heavy nucleus splits to form two lighter nuclei
D. a neutron breaks up a heavy nucleus
REF: 1-p. 70

498. Fission is the process whereby
A. two light nuclei coalesce to form a heavy nucleus
B. radium decays to radon
C. a heavy nucleus splits into two lighter nuclei
D. an a-particle is emitted from uranium
REF: 12-p. 119

499. Fission may be ____________ or ____________.
A. spontaneous; induced
B. spontaneous; primary
C. secondary; primary
D. secondary; induced
REF: 12-p. 119

500. When fission takes place, ____________ are released.
A. neutrons
B. alpha particles
C. protons
D. positrons
REF: 1-p. 69

501. The nuclear reactor is an example of controlled
A. fusion
B. fission
C. beta-minus-decay
D. beta-plus-decay
REF: 12-p. 119

502. The fuel for most nuclear reactors is composed of ____________ and/or ____________.
A. uranium; radium
B. radium; radon
C. uranium; plutonium
D. plutonium; radium
REF: 3-p. 69

503. In an (n, λ) reaction, the product is always an ________ of the target.
A. isotope
B. isotone
C. isobar
D. isomer
REF: 1-p. 71

504. The most common way of obtaining a short-lived daughter from a long-lived parent is
A. a nuclear reactor
B. a medical cyclotron
C. a radionuclide generator
D. direct air shipment
REF: 12-p. 133

505. In a radionuclide generator, the radioactive material is absorbed on a(n) ____________ exchange column.
A. alpha
B. beta minus
C. positron
D. ion
REF: 1-p. 69

506. The most commonly used ^{99}Mo--^{99m}Tc generator is the ____________ generator.
A. solvent extraction
B. sublimination
C. Alumina column
D. MEK
REF: 5 Vol. IV-p. 260

507. The equilibrium that would be established in a ^{99}Mo--^{99m}Tc generator if it were allowed to come to equilibrium is called ____________ equilibrium.
A. secular
B. permanent
C. chemical
D. transient
REF: 12-p. 45

508. When a ^{99}Mo generator is eluted the ^{99m}Tc is in the form of
A. TcO_5
B. TcO_{4+}
C. TcO_4^-
D. TcO_3^-
REF: 5 Vol. IV- p. 270

509. In order to bind Tc to phosphorus-oxygen compounds for bone scanning the Tc must be
A. oxidized to Tc (IV)
B. reduced to Tc (IV)
C. oxidized to Tc (VII)
D. reduced to Tc (VII)
REF: 5 Vol. IV-p. 274

510. The eluate of ^{99}Mo--^{99m}Tc generators should be checked for the presence of ^{99}Mo
A. each time a new generator is used
B. each day
C. each time the generator is eluted
D. each time a patient dose is prepared
REF: 12-p. 133

511. The concentration of ^{99}Mo in ^{99m}Tc shall not exceed
A. 0.5 µCi/mCi
B. 1 µCi/mCi
C. 2 µCi/mCi
D. 5 µCi/mCi
REF: 12-p. 133

512. Each patient dose of ^{99m}Tc shall not contain more than ____________ µCi of ^{99}Mo.
A. 1
B. 2
C. 5
D. 10
REF: 12-p. 133

513. A ^{99}Mo--^{99m}Tc generator is eluted at 8:00 a.m. Fifty µCi of ^{99}Mo is found in 200 mCi of ^{99m}Tc. Can this material be used to prepare a 15 mCi dose of ^{99m}Tc for brain scanning?
A. Yes
B. No
REF: 12-p. 133

514. Assuming the same conditions as the previous questions, could this material be used to prepare the 15 mCi dose at 3:00 p.m.?
A. Yes
B. No
REF: 12-p. 133

515. The limit of aluminum in the eluate of ^{99}Mo generator is
A. 20 µg/ml for fission ^{99}Mo
B. 20 µg/ml for reaction ^{99}Mo
C. 10 µg/ml for reaction ^{99}Mo
D. A and B
REF: 5 Vol. IV–p. 275

516. ____________ purity is the fraction of the stated radionuclide present in the stated chemical form.
A. Radioisotopic
B. Radionuclidic
C. Radiochemical
D. Radiopharmaceutical
REF: 10–p. 611

517. ____________ purity is the proportion of total activity present as the stated radionuclide.
A. Radioisotopic
B. Radionuclidic
C. Radiochemical
D. Radiopharmaceutical
REF: 10–p. 611

518. Mo–99 in the eluate of ^{99}Mo—^{99m}Tc generator is an example of a ____________ impurity.
A. radioisotopic
B. radionuclidic
C. radiochemical
D. radiopharmaceutical
REF: 10–p. 611

519. Free ^{131}I in a ^{131}I-triolein capsule is an example of a ____________ impurity.
A. radioisotopic
B. radionuclidic
C. radiochemical
D. radiopharmaceutical
REF: 10–p. 611

520. The concentration (C) of a radiopharmaceutical is given by
A. C = activity x volume
B. C = activity/volume
C. C = volume/activity
D. none of the above
REF: 1-p. 83

521. A vial contains 250 μCi of ^{75}Se in 5 ml of fluid. The concentration is
A. 250 μCi/ml
B. 50 μCi/ml
C. 5 μCi/ml
D. 1/5 μCi/ml
REF: 1-p. 82

522. The appropriate formula for determining the volume (V) required for a dose of activity (A) with a concentration (C) is
A. V = C/A
B. V = C x A
C. V = A/C
D. none of the above
REF: 1-p. 82

523. A vial contains ^{99m}Tc at a concentration of 58 mCi/ml. A dose of 15 mCi is desired. How many ml should be withdrawn into the syringe?
A. 0.87
B. 0.63
C. 0.38
D. 0.26
REF: 1-p. 82

524. A vial contains 350 mCi of ^{99m}Tc in 30 ml of fluid. What is the concentration?
A. 1050 mCi/ml
B. 105 mCi/ml
C. 85.7 mCi/ml
D. 11.67 mCi/ml
REF: 1-p. 119

525. A vial contains 385 μCi of ^{57}Co in 3 ml of fluid. What is the concentration?
A. 1155 μCi/ml
B. 128 μCi/ml
C. 77.9 μCi/ml
D. 55.4 μCi/ml
REF: 59–p. 119

526. How many ml should be withdrawn from the vial (previous question) to obtain 100 μCi?
A. 1.81
B. 1.28
C. 0.78
D. 0.09
REF: 59–p. 119

527. How many ml should be withdrawn from the vial (previous question) to obtain 23 mCi?
A. 1.97
B. 0.27
C. 0.22
D. 0.022
REF: 59–p. 119

528. Eighteen millicuries in 10 ml is added to 100 ml. The concentration is
A. 180 μCi/ml
B. 164 μCi/ml
C. 18 μCi/ml
D. 1.64 μCi/ml
REF: 59–p. 124

529. A ^{57}Co capsule is dissolved and water is added to make 100 ml. Ten ml are withdrawn and added to a bottle which is then filled to 1000 ml. The bottle is then counted and the results are compared with 1000 ml of urine in a similar bottle. This is an example of a ____________ standard.
A. 10%
B. 1%
C. 0.1%
D. 0.01%
REF: 59–p. 116

530. An ^{125}I capsule, similar to one given to a patient, is dissolved and water is added to make 50 ml. How many ml should be withdrawn to make a 5% standard?
A. 25
B. 10
C. 5
D. 2.5
REF: 59-p. 118

531. Radiation dose calculations are usually done using the
A. absolute activity model
B. absorbed fraction method
C. gamma--beta ratio model
D. pharmaceutical energy method
REF: 2 Suppl. 1-p. 9

532. Which of the following is not a factor in calculating radiation dose?
A. Concentration and duration of the radiopharmaceutical
B. Energy emitted by the pharmaceutical
C. Fraction of the emitted energy which is absorbed
D. All the above are used
REF: 2 Suppl. 1-p. 9

533. In doing radiopharmaceutical dose calculation for adults, a ____________ kg man is assumed.
A. 50
B. 70
C. 80
D. 90
REF: 2 Suppl. 3-p. 8

534. The absorbed fraction for beta-particles, when the target and source organs are the same, is
A. 0
B. 0.5
C. 1
D. 2
REF: 2 Suppl. 1-p. 12

535. The biologic half-life (Tb) is the time required for the body to eliminate, by its regular process, one-half of any ____________ substance.
A. stable
B. radioactive
C. either A or B
D. neither A nor B
REF: 1-p. 60

536. The appropriate formula for effective half-life (T_e) is
A. $T_e = \frac{T_p \times T_b}{T_p + T_b}$
B. $T_e = \frac{T_p + T_b}{T_p \times T_b}$
C. $Te = \frac{T_p \times T_b}{T_p - T_b}$
D. none of the ahove
REF: 1-p. 61

537. The effective half-life can never be longer than the
A. biological half-life
B. physical half-life
C. either A or B
D. neither A nor B
REF: 1-p. 61

538. If T_b = 26 hours and T_e = 18 hours, T_p =
A. 24 hours
B. 46 hours
C. 50 hours
D. 59 hours
REF: 1-p. 61

539. If T_e = 2.4 hours and T_p = 6 hours, T_b =
A. 2 hours
B. 4 hours
C. 6 hours
D. 10 hours
REF: 1-p. 61

540. If T_p = 8 days and T_b = 6 days, T_e =
A. 3.4 days
B. 4.3 days
C. 5.4 days
D. 14 days
REF: 1-p. 95

541. If T_b = 15 minutes and T_p = 6 hours, T_e =
A. 8.6 minutes
B. 14.4 minutes
C. 3.4 hours
D. 4.2 hours
REF: 1-p. 61

DIRECTIONS: The group of questions below consists of a list of lettered headings followed by a list of numbered words or statements. For **each** numbered word or statement, select the **one** lettered heading that is most closely associatsed with it. Each lettered heading may be selected once, more than once, or not at all.

IN THE REACTION A (b,c) D:

A. Bombarding radiation
B. Released radiation
C. Target nucleus
D. Product nucleus

542. A = ____________

543. B = ____________

544. C = ____________

545. D = ____________

REF: 1-p. 71

10. HEMATOLOGY

DIRECTIONS: Each of the questions or incomplete statements below is followed by a list of suggested answers or completions. Select the **one** that is **BEST** in each case.

---

546. All of the following are plasma proteins EXCEPT
A. globulins
B. albumin
C. fibrinogen
D. hormones
REF: 36-p. 269

547. The average hemoglobin content of the blood in an adult is
A. 15 gm/100 ml
B. 45 gm/100 ml
C. 12 gm/100 ml
D. 10 gm/100 ml
REF: 1-p. 346; 37-p. 270

548. The fluid portion of an uncoagulated blood sample is called
A. plasma
B. serum
REF: 1-p. 345

549. The life of a red blood cell in man spans
A. 10 days
B. 30 days
C. 60 days
D. 120 days
REF: 1-p. 346

550. Which element is essential in the synthesis of hemoglobin?
A. Iodine
B. Selenium
C. Chromium
D. Iron
REF: 1-p. 346

551. All of the following are types of white blood cells EXCEPT
A. thrombocytes
B. granulocytes
C. lymphocytes
D. monocytes
REF: 1-p. 346

552. Neutrophils, eosinophils, and basophils are all types of
A. lymphocytes
B. thrombocytes
C. monocytes
D. granulocytes
REF: 1-p. 346

553. The plasma protein which functions in blood clotting is
A. albumin
B. alpha globulin
C. gamma globulin
D. fibrinogen
REF: 1-p. 345

554. One of the primary functions of platelets is to
A. combat infections
B. develop immunities
C. form a hemostatic plug after injury
D. produce antibodies
REF: 1-p. 346

555. The volume of packed erythrocytes expressed as a percentage of the blood sample is called the
A. mean blood volumc
B. plasmacrit
C. hematocrit
D. red cell count
REF: 1-p. 345

556. The average value for a normal hematocrit is approximately
A. 25%
B. 35%
C. 45%
D. 55%
REF: 1-p. 345; 37-p. 269

557. Serum differs from plasma primarily in that it contains no
A. prothrombin
B. gamma globulins
C. fibrinogen
D. red blood cells
REF: 1-p. 345

558. In a spun anticoagulated blood sample, the layer of cells directly above the red cells is composed of
A. platelets
B. white blood cells
C. immunoglobulins
D. lipoproteins
REF: 32-p. 403

559. The hematocrit value of a given blood sample represents
A. the ratio between the plasma compartment and the cellular compartment
B. the ratio between the serum compartment and the cellular compartment
C. the percentage of the various components of the blood
D. the ratio of the red blood cells to white blood cells
REF: 32-p. 403

560. What is the effect of dehydration upon the hematocrit of the patient?
A. It falsely elevates the hematocrit
B. It falsely lowers the hematocrit
C. It does not affect the hematocrit reading
REF: 32-p. 404

561. The dilution principle is used in all of the following procedures EXCEPT
A. plasma volume
B. thyroid uptake
C. red cell volume
D. body water
REF: 35-p. 148

562. The dilution principle can be expressed mathematically as
A. $Q = V \times C$
B. $V = Q \times C$
C. $V = \frac{Q \times C}{2}$
D. $\frac{V}{2} = Q \times C$
REF: 36-p. 270

563. Radiotracers used in dilution studies, i.e., blood volume determinations, should exhibit all of the following characteristics EXCEPT
A. the radiotracer should have a high keV energy for better counting statistics
B. the radiotracer should not alter the normal physiologic processes in the body
C. the radiotracer should behave in a manner which is identical to the parent compound being studied
D. the tracer should be nontoxic
REF: 35-p. 147

564. Radionuclides used for blood volume determination may either be tagged to plasma proteins or to the
A. serum
B. white blood cells
C. platelets
D. erythrocytes
REF: 36-p. 271

565. Red cell volume determination is useful in patients with
A. anemia
B. hypertension
C. vitamin C deficiency
D. polycythemia vera
E. A, B, and C only
F. A, B, and D only
REF: 36-p. 283

566. A normal 70 kg adult male should have a total blood volume of approximately
A. 2000 ml
B. 3080 ml
C. 4620 ml
D. 5040 ml
REF: 1-p. 351

567. The most common radioactive tagging agent used in red cell volume determinations is
A. ^{125}I HSA
B. ^{131}I HSA
C. ^{51}Cr chromic chloride
D. ^{51}Cr sodium chromate
REF: 1-p. 349

568. The principal gamma energy and half-life (T_p) of ^{51}Cr is
A. 122 keV, 270 days
B. 810 keV, 71.3 days
C. 320 keV, 27.8 days
D. 412 keV, 2.7 days
REF: 36-p. 584

569. The form(s) of ^{51}Cr which can permeate the red cell membrane is (are)
A. the trivalent form
B. the bivalent form
C. the hexavalent form
D. all of the above
REF: 36-p. 275

570. The rate of ^{51}Cr sodium chromate binding to the red cell varies with
A. temperature
B. pH
C. the age of the red blood cell
D. all of the above
E. A and B only
REF: 37-p. 381

571. Exogenous substances in patients which interfere with the tagging action of ^{51}Cr sodium chromate by acting as reducing agents include
A. antibiotics
B. polyvitamins
C. pain medications
D. A and B only
E. all of the above
REF: 32-p. 288

572. The action of ACD solution is as
A. a cell preserver
B. a pH stabilizer
C. a reducing agent
D. an anticoagulant
REF: 36-p. 286

573. The ratio of ACD solution to whole blood used in blood volume determinations is
A. 1:1
B. 1:2
C. 1:5
D. 1:10
REF: 37-p. 377

574. Which portion of the ACD solution acts as a reducing agent, thereby prohibiting addition of ^{51}Cr sodium chromate to the solution before the addition of the whole blood?
A. Citric acid
B. Sodium citrate
C. Dextrose
D. Heparin
REF: 36-p. 288

575. The purpose of adding ascorbic acid to the ACD-whole-blood-^{51}Cr mixture in red blood cell volume determinations is to

A. stimulate the tagging action of the radiochromate
B. increase permeability of the red cell membrane
C. isolate the hemoglobin portion of the blood
D. reduce the hexavalent radiochromate to the trivalent state
REF: 36-p. 275

576. Care should be taken in red cell volume determination not to hemolyze the red blood cells because

A. the red cell volume will be superficially low
B. the red cell volume will be superficially high
C. the hematocrit will be markedly high
D. the plasmacrit will be markedly low
REF: 32-p. 408

577. Hemolysis of the blood sample can occur as a result of

A. rapid withdrawal and injection of the sample
B. frothing of the blood in the syringe
C. using a needle with a high gauge number
D. excessive shaking of the sample
E. A, B, and C only
F. all of the above
REF: 42-p. 105

578. The purpose of injecting the tracer and obtaining the subsequent samples from opposite arms in blood volume determinations is to

A. lessen the chances of extravasation
B. give the patient's arm a rest
C. use one arm for the red cell volume and the opposite arm for plasma volume
D. avoid contamination of residual tracer left at injection site
REF: 32-p. 272

579. To insure complete mixing of the tracer with the patient's blood, the first sample should be taken ________ minutes after injection of the tracer.
A. 2
B. 10
C. 30
D. 45
REF: 36-p. 272

580. Delayed mixing of the labeled blood and circulating blood during a red cell volume determination occurs in patients with
A. splenomegaly
B. acute blood loss
C. severe polycythemia
D. bone marrow disturbances
E. all of the above
F. A and C only
REF: 32-p. 407

581. Extravasation of the tracer during performance of a blood volume determination will result in calculations which are
A. superficially high
B. superficially low
C. unaffected by this factor
REF: 32-p. 408

582. A hematocrit correction factor of 0.89 is necessary in blood volume determinations calculations because of
A. differences occurring in hematocrits obtained form different-sized vessels
B. differences occurring in hematocrits of different organs
C. variations due to plasma trapped in cells during hematocrit determinations
D. all of the above
REF: 1-p. 347

583. If the patient's own blood is unavailable for blood volume determinations, which of the following may be used as an alternative?
A. Group O, Rh^- blood
B. Group A, Rh^+ blood
C. Synthetic red blood cells
D. The patient's own blood *must* be used
REF: 36-p. 277

584. Spuriously elevated results during red cell volume determinations are caused by all of the following EXCEPT
A. extravasation of the injected dose
B. hemolysis of the sample
C. abnormally high levels of leukocytes or platelets
D. previously administered radionuclides
REF: 32-p. 408

585. The normal plasma volume for a 70 kg adult male is approximately
A. 2000 ml
B. 3080 ml
C. 4000 ml
D. 5040 ml
REF: 1-p. 351

586. The radiotracer used in plasma volume determinations tags onto which portion of the plasma?
A. Inorganic constituents
B. Hormones
C. Amino acids
D. Plasma proteins
REF: 1-p. 347

587. All of the following have been used to label plasma proteins for plasma volume determinations EXCEPT
A. ^{131}I HSA
B. ^{125}I HSA
C. ^{51}Cr sodium chromate
D. ^{113m}In chloride
REF: 36-p. 271

588. A common tracer which is used in blood volume tests and which tags the plasma portion of blood is
A. ^{125}I human serum albumin
B. ^{51}Cr-sodium
C. ^{131}I-hippuran
D. ^{75}Se-methionine
REF: 36-p. 408

589. The principal gamma energy and half-life of ^{125}I is
A. 159 keV, 13 hours
B. 364 keV, 8.08 days
C. 173 keV, 2.8 days
D. 35 keV, 60 days
REF: 36-p. 584

590. The purpose of multiple sampling at sequential time intervals in plasma volume determination is to
A. decrease the chance of error from any one sample
B. establish the rate of leak-out of the albumin from the vascular system
C. account for physical decay of the radionuclide
D. extract as much radioactivity as possible from the patient to reduce exposure
REF: 32-p. 272

591. Which factor(s) may interfere with correct plasma volume measurements?
A. Recent exercise
B. Climatic conditions
C. Pregnancy
D. B and C only
E. All of the above
REF: 35-p. 205

592. In a red cell survival study, the normal disappearance half-time is approximately
A. 10-15 days
B. 25-35 days
C. 40-60 days
D. 110-120 days
REF: 1-p. 353

593. In a red cell survival determination, the daily percent values are plotted on log-linear paper against
A. hematocrit values
B. corrected daily percent values
C. time lapse in days
D. daily count rates
REF: 36-p. 294

594. ^{51}Cr sodium chromate, when used as a random label, binds to
A. thrombocytes
B. white blood cells
C. albumin
D. red blood cells
E. all of the above
F. A, B, and D only
REF: 31-p. 217

595. In a red cell survival study, a waiting period of 24 hours between injection of the radiolabeled blood and taking the first sample is necessary
A. to allow for removal from the circulation of any cells damaged during the labeling procedure
B. to allow the ^{51}Cr to tag permanently to the hemoglobin
C. to prevent contamination of samples at the injection site
D. all of the above
E. A and C only
REF: 32-p. 409

596. In a red cell survival determination, samples are taken from the patient
A. every day for 1 week
B. every other day for 3 weeks
C. every other week for 1 month
D. every week for 1 month
REF: 32-p. 409

597. All samples of a red cell survival study are counted at the same time after the final sample has been collected to

A. allow the radioactive ^{51}Cr to tag permanently to the hemoglobin
B. allow for complete mixing of the radiolabeled blood and the patient's blood
C. abolish the effects of physical decay of the radio-nuclide
D. save time and money for the patient

REF: 1-p. 353

598. The main difference between red blood cells labeled by the cohort method and those labeled by the random method is

A. the number of cells labeled
B. the ages of the cells labeled
C. the location of the label
D. none

REF: 32-p. 406

599. The selective or cohort labeling technique used in red cell survival studies is

A. the method of choice due to its simplicity
B. the method most frequently used in the study of erythrocyte survival
C. seldom used due to its expense and a long period of observation
D. never used because erythrocytes of identical age are impossible to isolate

REF: 1-p. 352

600. Disadvantages of the random labeling method for red cell survival studies include all of the following EXCEPT

A. wide fluctuations in the blood volume may invalidate the results
B. inability to differentiate a short finite life-span from random destruction of red cells
C. the accuracy in percentages decreases toward the latter end of the study
D. the length of time needed to complete the study may approach 4 months

REF: 1-p. 352

601. In a red cell survival determination, an extracorpuscular abnormality can be detected using
A. donor cells
B. patient's own cells
—**C.** both of the above
D. none of the above
REF: 37-p. 387

602. A source(s) of error which may falsely alter the results in a red cell survival determination is (are)
A. blood transfusion during study
B. increased fluid intake during study
C. decreased fluid intake during study
D. acute blood loss during the study
E. all of the above
—**F.** A and D only
REF: 32-p. 410

603. A markedly shortened red cell survival half-time may be indicative of which disease process(es)?
A. Polycythemia vera
B. Hypersplenism
C. Hemolytic anemia
D. All of the above
—**E.** B and C only
REF: 31-p. 219; 34-p. 240

604. Which of the following conditions occurring during the study period may affect and skew the red cell survival curve?
A. Active blood loss
B. Transfusions
C. Increased red cell production
—**D.** All of the above
E. A and B only
REF: 33-p. 240

605. Studies which can be done concurrently with a red cell survival study include
- **A.** red cell volume
- **B.** splenic sequestration study
- **C.** liver/spleen scintigraphy
- **D.** enteric blood loss study
- **E.** all of the above
- **F.** A, B, and D

REF: 32-p. 410

606. The purpose of a splenic sequestration study using ^{51}Cr labeled red blood cells is to
- **A.** ascertain splenomegaly
- **B.** determine sites of increased red blood cell destruction
- **C.** determine sites of red blood cell storage
- **D.** determine sites of erythropoiesis

REF: 36-p. 294

607. Body sites which are externally counted on the patient every other day in a splenic sequestration study are the
- **A.** liver, spleen, and bladder
- **B.** liver, spleen, and manubrium
- **C.** liver, spleen, and precordium
- **D.** liver, spleen, and sacrum

REF: 36-p. 294

608. The normal spleen-to-liver ratio in a splenic sequestration study is approximately
- **A.** 1:1
- **B.** 2:1
- **C.** 1:2
- **D.** 3:1

REF: 36-p. 294

609. Of the body's total iron, about 60% is contained in
- **A.** porphyrin rings
- **B.** bilirubin and biliverdin pigments
- **C.** the bone marrow
- **D.** the hemoglobin of the red blood cells

REF: 37-p. 166

610. Total body iron content averages
A. 4.5 mg
B. 12.5 mg
C. 4.5 gm
D. 12.5 gm
REF: 1-p. 356

611. Iron loss, which occurs as a result of blood loss, body secretions, urine and bile excretions, averages approximately ____________ per day.
A. 0.5–1.5 μg
B. 2–3 μg
C. 0.5–1.5 mg
D. 2–3 mg
REF: 1-p. 357

612. Absorption of dietary iron, of which only about 10% is absorbed, takes place mainly in the
A. large intestine
B. stomach
C. duodenum
D. cecum
REF: 1-p. 356

613. After its absorption from the gut, iron is then carried in the plasma by way of
A. gamma globulins
B. albumin
C. transferrin
D. hormones
REF: 32-p. 411

614. The normal half-time plasma iron clearance rate using ^{59}Fe ferrous citrate is between
A. 0–1 hours
B. 1–2 hours
C. 2–4 hours
D. 4–6 hours
REF: 36-p. 297

615. In plasma iron clearance half-time test, the activity of blood samples is plotted on
A. linear-linear paper vs time (in minutes)
B. linear-linear paper vs iron half-life (in days)
C. log-linear paper vs iron clearance (in minutes)
D. log-linear paper vs time (in minutes)
REF: 36-p. 298

616. Half-time plasma iron clearance rates are shortened in
A. aplastic anemia
B. hemolytic anemia
C. hemochromatosis
D. polycythemia vera
E. all of the above
F. B and D only
REF: 36-p. 297

617. Prolonged plasma iron turnover rates (PITR) are seen in
A. polycythemia vera
B. hemolytic anemia
C. aplastic anemia
D. blood loss
REF: 36-p. 298

618. The normal range for plasma iron turnover rate is
A. 0.1-0.5 mg/24 hr
B. 12-15 mg/24 hr
C. 27-42 mg/24 hr
D. 63-75 mg/24 hr
REF: 36-p. 299

619. Iron utilization rates are accelerated in
A. hemolytic anemia
B. polycythemia vera
C. pernicious anemia
D. all of the above
E. A and B only
REF: 36-p. 299

620. Plasma iron turnover rates may be used as an index of
A. blood volume
B. hemoglobin measurement
C. erythropoietic activity
D. hemosiderin formation
REF: 1-p. 357

621. Heparin is the anticoagulant of choice when collecting blood samples for iron metabolism studies because
A. it enhances uptake of the radioiron by transferrin
B. it will not chelate the iron as other anticoagulants may
C. it strengthens the bond between the transferrin and radioiron
D. it prevents elution loss of the radioiron into the body tissues
REF: 32-p. 412

622. Surface counting to determine organ localization of ^{59}Fe is generally done over which of the following areas?
A. Liver, spleen, spine, precordium
B. Liver, spleen, sternum, precordium
C. Liver, spleen, femoral head, precordium
D. Liver, spleen, sacrum, precordium
REF: 32-p. 413

623. The radioactive isotope of iron currently used in iron metabolism studies is
A. ^{57}Fe
B. ^{26}Fe
C. ^{55}Fe
D. ^{59}Fe
REF: 1-p. 357

624. Low red cell utilization rates of radioiron are seen in
A. polycythemia vera
B. iron deficiency anemia
C. pernicious anemia
D. all of the above
REF: 37-p. 169

625. In a normal radioiron distribution study, early peaking at 2 days post injection, then a rapid decrease in activity would likely occur over the
A. sacrum
B. precordium
C. liver
D. spleen
REF: 1-p. 358

626. In a normal radioiron distribution study, peak activity occurring 7-10 days after injection over the precordial area represents
A. radioiron which is not transferrin-bound
B. radioiron which is tagged to the myocardium
C. newly formed erythrocytes in the circulating blood
D. extramedullary erythropoiesis
REF: 1-p. 358

627. In normal subjects, 60-80% of an administered radioiron dose will be incorporated into circulating erythrocytes in
A. 2-5 days
B. 7-10 days
C. 15-20 days
D. 20-30 days
REF: 32-p. 413

628. The most common cause of vitamin B_{12} malabsorption is
A. drug therapy with PAS
B. small bowel blind loops
C. pancreatic insufficiency
D. deficiency in intrinsic factor
REF: 32-p. 414

629. Intrinsic factor is a glycoprotein secreted by the
A. jejunum
B. stomach
C. duodenum
D. ileum
REF: 32-p. 414

630. Dietary vitamin B_{12}, in the presence of intrinsic factor, is normally absorbed in the
A. jejunum
B. stomach
C. duodenum
D. ileum
REF: 32-p. 414

631. The organ system(s) most profoundly affected by vitamin B_{12} deficiency is (are)
A. bone marrow
B. genitourinary system
C. gastrointestinal system
D. neurologic system
E. all of the above
F. A, C, and D only
REF: 36-p. 259

632. Possible causes of a vitamin B_{12} deficiency are
A. failure of the stomach to secrete intrinsic factor
B. defect in absorption
C. intraintestinal bacterial destruction of vitamin B_{12}
D. all of the above
REF: 36-p. 259

633. Failure to absorb dietary vitamin B_{12} will eventually lead to
A. pernicious anemia
B. microcytic anemia
C. leukemia
D. hyperchromic anemia
REF: 36-p. 259

634. Vitamin B_{12}, which is not stored in the body, is excreted primarily via the
A. urine
B. feces
C. bile
D. all of the above
REF: 32-p. 415

635. Absorption of vitamin B_{12} can be studied by one or more of the following tests
A. fecal excretion
B. plasma radioactivity
C. hepatic uptake
D. urinary excretion
E. all of the above
F. B and D only
REF: 1-p. 359

636. In the Schilling test, an oral dose of tagged vitamin B_{12} is followed by a parenteral dose of nonlabeled B_{12}. Samples of ____________ are then collected and counted.
A. feces
B. blood
C. plasma
D. urine
REF: 14-p. 642

637. Patient preparations for the Schilling test include all of the following EXCEPT
A. overnight fast
B. flushing dose of a diuretic
C. oral and parenteral vitamin B_{12} held prior to test
D. background urine sample
REF: 32-p. 414

638. A factor(s) which may interfere with the results of a Schilling test is (are)
A. vitamin B_{12} injections
B. colchicine corticosteroids
C. fasting
D. A and B only
E. A and C only
REF: 32-p. 414

639. The time interval between administration of the tagged vitamin B_{12} and the "flushing" dose of "cold" vitamin B_{12} is

A. 20 minutes
B. 2 hours
C. 12 hours
D. 2 days
REF: 36-p. 260

640. The purpose of administering a "flushing" dose of 1000 μg of nonradioactive vitamin B_{12} when performing a Schilling test is

A. to increase ileal absorption of the radioactive B_{12}
B. to achieve transient saturation of normal binding sites in plasma
C. to stimulate the gastric mucosa to secrete intrinsic factor
D. to reduce the radioactive B_{12} to a nonabsorptive state
REF: 33-p. 242

641. If the flushing dose of nonradioactive B_{12} is *not* given when performing a Schilling test, the results would be

A. erroneously normal
B. erroneously low
C. erroneously high
D. unaffected
REF: 33-p. 243

642. The dose of ^{57}Co-vitamin B_{12} given for a Schilling test is generally

A. 0.5 μCi
B. 5.0 μCi
C. 50 μCi
D. 500 μCi
REF: 32-p. 415

643. If the urinary excretion of ^{57}Co-B_{12} is less than 7%, the test is usually repeated except the labeled vitamin is administered with

A. hog intrinsic factor
B. vitamin C
C. antibiotics
D. lasix
REF: 1-p. 361

644. A value of 5% (of the administered dose) is calculated on a Schilling test done without intrinsic factor. This could be caused by

A. malabsorption of vitamin B_{12}
B. renal disease
C. incomplete urine collection
D. all of the above
E. none of the above
REF: 32-p. 415

645. A patient has had two Schilling tests performed on him. The first result was 3%. The second result, performed with intrinsic factor, was 14%. This patient probably has

A. pancreatic insufficiency
B. Zollinger-Ellison syndrome
C. regional ileitis
D. pernicious anemia
REF: 32-p. 415

646. Currently, it is possible to simultaneously evaluate vitamin B_{12} absorption with and without intrinsic factor using which radionuclides?

A. ^{57}Co and ^{60}Co
B. ^{57}Co and ^{58}Co
C. ^{58}Co and ^{60}Co
D. ^{58}Co and ^{59}Co
REF: 33-p. 242

647. In a patient with pernicious anemia, the urinary excretion of labeled vitamin B_{12}, when administered with the hog intrinsic factor, will
A. decrease to near zero
B. decrease to abnormal values
C. increase
D. remain the same
REF: 1-p. 361

648. One source of error in the Schilling test may be
A. reabsorption of the radio-cobalt label
B. incomplete collection of fecal sample
C. incomplete collection of urine samples
D. contamination of the feces with urine
REF: 33-p. 243

649. The bone marrow may be imaged using radiopharmaceuticals which are taken up by the
A. reticuloendothelial cells
B. erythrons
C. osteoblasts
D. all of the above
E. A and B only
REF: 31-p. 57

650. Bone marrow scanning can be used to
A. localize functional marrow
B. estimate the effects of bone irradiation
C. determine the rate of erythropoiesis
D. all of the above
E. A and B only
REF: 31-p. 59

651. Radiopharmaceuticals which have been used to image the bone marrow include all of the following EXCEPT
A. ^{113m}In colloid
B. ^{51}Cr sodium chromate
C. ^{99m}Tc sulfur colloid
D. ^{52}Fe
REF: 36-p. 488

652. Erythropoiesis in the normal adult occurs in the bone marrow of all of the following EXCEPT
A. distal humeri
B. vertebral column
C. pelvis
D. sternum
REF: 36-p. 489; 39-p. 242

653. Conditions which cause peripheral marrow expansion and consequent abnormal radionuclide marrow images include all of the following EXCEPT
A. iron deficiency anemia
B. polycythemia vera
C. chronic hemolytic anemia
D. acute hemolytic anemia
REF: 33-p. 247

654. Bone marrow scans are useful in evaluating patients with
A. aplastic anemia
B. polycythemia vera
C. metastatic disease
D. all of the above
E. A and B only
REF: 17-p. 126

655. Drawbacks to the use of ^{99m}Tc sulfur colloid in imaging bone marrow include all of the following EXCEPT
A. its uptake by the liver and spleen may obscure structures in those areas
B. its uptake by the RE cells of the marrow corresponds consistently with erythropoiesis only in normal cases
C. its preparation and availability do not lend themselves well to routine use
D. its proportionately low uptake in the bone marrow itself which results in larger doses as well as longer imaging times
REF: 38-p. 243

656. In addition to technical factors, the main source of error in plasma volume determinations is

A. leakage of the tracer from the vascular compartment
B. physical decay of the radionuclide
C. weak tag of the radiopharmaceutical
D. differences in hematocrits taken from various sampling sites
REF: 1-p. 348

657. Platelet survival studies are performed using ________ as the radiolabel.

A. ^{51}Cr sodium chromate
B. ^{75}Se selenomethionine
C. ^{59}Fe ferrous citrate
D. ^{99m}Tc sulfur colloid
REF: 1-p. 355

658. The normal life-span of platelets using the radiolabeling method is

A. 8-11 days
B. 25-35 days
C. 60-80 days
D. 120-130 days
REF: 1-p. 356

659. White cell survival studies can be performed using ____________ as the radiolabel.

A. ^{51}Cr sodium chromate
B. ^{111}In oxine
C. ^{99m}Tc sulfur colloid
D. all of the above
E. A and B only
REF: 1-p. 355

660. Red cell survival is used to determine the life span of erythrocytes in patients with

A. pernicious anemia
B. acute anemia
C. hemolytic anemia
D. erythroblastosis fetalis
REF: 36-p. 293

661. In a red cell survival study, the disappearance half-time represents the time after injection of the labeled erythrocytes at which the radioactivity in the blood level has fallen to ____________ of its initial value.

A. 25%

B. 50%

C. 75%

D. 100%

REF: 1-p. 353

11. RADIOIMMUNOASSAYS

DIRECTIONS: Each of the questions or incomplete statements below is followed by a list of suggested answers or completions. Select the **one** that is **BEST** in each case.

---

662. The principle of radioimmunoassay is based upon the fact that

A. both labeled and unlabeled antigens will combine to form a measurable entity

B. only labeled antibody and labeled antigen will combine to form a measurable entity

C. only unlabeled antigen will complex with the labeled antibody to form a measurable entity

D. both labeled and unlabeled antigen will complex with a known amount of antibody to form a measurable entity

REF: 1-p. 600

663. The term "radioimmunoassay" is synonymous with

A. saturation analysis

B. competitive-binding analysis

C. displacement analysis

D. all of the above

E. A and C only

REF: 32-p. 444

664. In general, the basic components of an RIA reaction are
A. labeled antibody, unlabeled antigen
B. antibody, labeled antigen
C. antibody, labeled antigen, unlabeled antigen
D. labeled antibody, unlabeled antibody, antigen
REF: 40-p. 49

665. The principle of equilibrium used in radioimmunoassay which states that, if a system is initially at equilibrium and is forced away from equilibrium when one parameter is changed, then the system will spontaneously return to a new equilibrium, is known as
A. Le Châtelier's principle
B. the mass action principle
C. the saturation principle
D. the law of constant composition
REF: 32-p. 445

666. A substance produced in response to an antigen that reacts specifically with that antigen is called
A. a hapten
B. an antibody
C. an adjuvant
D. an immunogen
REF: 1-p. 599

667. Antigens are also known as
A. antisera
B. antibodies
C. immunogens
D. haptens
REF: 1-p. 600

668. In general, a substance must have a molecular weight exceeding at least ____________ in order to be antigenic.
A. 5000
B. 10,000
C. 15,000
D. 20,000
REF: 32-p. 448

669. A substance that increases the formation and persistence of antibodies when injected together with antigens is called
A. an adjuvant
B. an antiserum
C. a hapten
D. a hormone
REF: 1-p. 598

670. The titer of the antibody is a term which refers most specifically to
A. avidity
B. affinity
C. concentration
D. stability
REF: 1-p. 601

671. The most important consideration regarding the antibody used in a radioimmunoassay procedure is
A. its affinity for the antigen
B. its titer or concentration
C. its final quantity
D. its source
REF: 39-p. 34

672. The affinity of a particular assay's antibody determines the ____________ of that assay.
A. avidity
B. specificity
C. sensitivity
D. accuracy
REF: 34-p. 33

673. In a radioimmunoassay system, the sensitivity of the assay is dependent on two factors relating to the labeled antigen. These are
A. that the radiolabel of the antigen be a beta-emitting radionuclide
B. that the labeled antigen react with the antibody in the same manner as the unlabeled antigen
C. that the labeled antigen be of a high specific activity
D. A and B
E. A and C
F. B and C
REF: 1-p. 607

674. The amount of radiolabeled antibody-antigen complex formed in a radioimmunoassay reaction is
A. directly dependent on the amount of unlabeled antigen present
B. directly dependent on the amount of labeled antibody present
C. inversely dependent on the amount of unlabeled antibody present
D. inversely dependent on the amount of unlabeled antigen present
REF: 32-p. 444

675. The extent to which a given measurement agrees with its actual value is termed
A. sensitivity
B. specificity
C. accuracy
D. precision
REF: 1-p. 598

676. Selectivity in radioimmunoassays can also be referred to as
A. sensitivity
B. specificity
C. precision
D. accuracy
REF: 32-p. 445

677. The sensitivity of a competitive-binding radioassay is partially determined by two related properties of the specific reactor substance. These are
A. affinity
B. avidity
C. accuracy
D. A and B only
E. A and C only
REF: 32-p. 445

678. The term "antibody" is synonymous with
A. antiserum
B. immunoglobulin
C. immunogen
D. all of the above
E. A and B only
F. B and C only
REF: 1-p. 610

679. In an RIA procedure, the material to be measured is referred to as the
A. antibody
B. immunoglobulin
C. specific reactor substance
D. ligand
REF: 32-p. 443

680. The purpose of having a nonspecific binding or "Blank" tube when performing an RIA procedure is to measure the amount of
A. nonspecific binding of the antibody
B. nonspecific binding of radioisotopic contamination
C. labeled antibody which is bound to unlabeled ligand
D. labeled ligand which is bound to nonspecific elements in the assay
REF: 40-p. 319

681. In radioimmunoassay procedures, the solutions of known antigen concentrations are called the
A. controls
B. nonspecific binding tubes
C. blanks
D. standards
REF: 1-p. 601

682. 10^{-12} gm equals one
A. picogram
B. nanogram
C. microgram
D. milligram
REF: 37-p. 454

683. Major advantages of radioimmunoassay techniques over other bioassays include:
A. it is highly specific
B. it is highly sensitive
C. it requires small volumes of sample fluid
D. all of the above
E. A and C only
REF: 37-p. 454

684. The binding reaction between antibody and antigen generally ____________ as the temperature increases, while its affinity ____________ as the temperature increases.
A. increases; increases
B. increases; decreases
C. decreases; decreases
D. decreases; increases
REF: 40-p. 61

685. The appearance of the binding curve in a competitive-binding equilibrium RIA is dependent on all of the following factors EXCEPT
A. the total antibody concentration
B. the affinity constant, K, of the antibody
C. the total labeled antigen concentration
D. the total number of standards
REF: 40-p. 61

686. The strength of an antibody-antigen reaction is expressed by the
A. law of mass action
B. Le Châtelier's principle
C. equilibrium constant
D. Berson-Yalow principle
REF: 40-p. 49

687. Advantages of using ^{125}I over ^{131}I as a radiolabel in RIA procedures include all of the following EXCEPT
A. it has a longer half-life
B. it allows higher counting efficiency
C. it has a higher specific activity
D. it is more stable
REF: 40-p. 52

688. The K value of an RIA equilibrium reaction can be influenced by all of the following EXCEPT
A. pH
B. temperature
C. ionic environment
D. patient status
E. all of the above
REF: 32-p. 445

689. What is the property of bioassays which demonstrates that the dilution curve of an elevated sample will match the standard curve for the assay by a constant factor and with linearity?
A. Accuracy
B. Parallelism
C. Precision
D. Recovery
REF: 40-p. 39

690. In kit evaluation techniques, percent recovery can be determined by the following equation
A. $\frac{\text{total analyte found}}{\text{total analyte expected}}$
B. $\frac{\text{total analyte added}}{\text{total analyte found}}$
C. $\frac{\text{total analyte recovered}}{\text{total analyte expected}}$
D. $\frac{\text{total analyte added}}{\text{total analyte expected}}$
REF: 40-p. 38

691. The serum sample size required for most RIA procedures ranges from
A. 0.1 to 5.0 µl
B. 10 to 200 µl
C. 300 to 500 µl
D. 1000 to 2000 µl
REF: 40-p. 36

692. Precision, intraassay or interassay, is usually calculated using which statistical measure?
A. Percent coefficient of variation
B. Analysis of variance
C. Standard deviation
D. Correlation coefficient
REF: 40-p. 37

693. The property of antisera whereby antibodies react with two or more antigens of similar structure and which reduces the specificity of the assay is known as
A. sensitivity
B. cross-reactivity
C. avidity
D. antigenicity
REF: 32-p. 448

694. All of the following are methods of radioiodination used in preparation of highly purified radioiodinated proteins and peptides EXCEPT
A. chloramine-T
B. water-soluble carbodiimide
C. lactoperoxidase
D. Bolton-Hunter
REF: 34-p. 70

695. The isotope most commonly used in RIA procedures is
A. ^{131}I
B. ^{14}C
C. ^{3}H
D. ^{125}I
REF: 34-p. 71

696. Chromatoelectrophoresis, solid-phase, double-antibody immunoprecipitation, filtration, and centrifugation are all methods used to
A. iodinate the labeled antigen
B. separate bound from free antigen
C. purify the labeled antigen
D. produce antibodies for use in the assay
REF: 40-p. 65

697. All of the following methods have been used to separate bound from free analyte EXCEPT
A. gel filtration
B. polymerized antibodies
C. lactoperoxidase
D. immunoprecipitation
REF: 34–p. 108

698. All of the following are reagents used in chemical separation methods EXCEPT
A. ethanol
B. polyethylene glycol
C. trichloracetic acid
D. Sephadex
REF: 34–p. 115

699. Separation of bound from free analyte using cross-linked dextrans such as Sephadex columns is known as
A. gel filtration
B. immunoprecipitation
C. chemical separation
D. adsorbent separation
REF: 34–p. 110

700. Immunoprecipitation, a type of separation technique used in RIA procedures, is also known as
A. gel filtration
B. Sephadex separation
C. double antibody technique
D. adsorbent methodology
REF: 34–p. 110

701. In data reduction methods for RIA procedures, plotting of the data on a ____________ scale produces a curved line, whereas use of a ____________ scale produces a straight line.
A. linear–linear; log–linear
B. log–logit; log–linear
C. linear–linear; log–logit
D. all of the above
E. A and C only
REF: 40–p. 320

702. The Scatchard plot, introduced for RIA by Berson and Yalow, is used in estimating
A. the specificity of the assay
B. the accuracy of the assay
C. the equilibrium constant of the assay
D. the reciprocity of the assay
REF: 40-p. 76

703. Cortisol, a glucocorticosteroid, is secreted by the part of the adrenal gland known as the
A. medulla
B. glomerulosa
C. zona fasciculata
D. zona reticularis
REF: 40-p. 119

704. Which of the following anterior pituitary hormones controls the secretion of cortisol from the adrenal cortex?
A. ADH
B. ACTH
C. FSH
D. GH
REF: 40-p. 119

705. A cortisol level which is drawn in the early a.m. will be ____________ than a level which was drawn the evening before.
A. greater than
B. less than
C. the same as
REF: 40-p. 119

706. Transient hypercortisolism may be caused by
A. hyperglycemia
B. hypoglycemia
C. drug-induced sleep
D. edema
REF: 40-p. 120

707. Cushing's syndrome, which can be caused by adrenal hyperplasia, is often characterized by ___________ levels of cortisol.
A. elevated
B. diminished
C. unchanged
REF: 40-p. 123

708. Elevated cortisol levels which are suppressible after the administration of dexamethasone are indicative of
A. Addison's disease
B. ACTH secreting carcinoma
C. autonomous adrenal tumor
D. Cushing's disease
REF: 40-p. 124

709. ACTH stimulation tests, used in conjunction with plasma cortisol levels, are of clinical utility in differentiation of
A. Addison's from Cushing's disease
B. pituitary insufficiency from Cushing's disease
C. pituitary insufficiency from Addison's disease
D. adrenal hyperplasia from adrenal tumor
REF: 36-p. 316

710. Radioimmunoassay procedures have proven useful in detection of all of the following hepatitis B markers EXCEPT
A. Anti-HBc
B. Anti-HBe
C. HBs Ag
D. HBc Ag
E. All of the above can be detected by RIA methodology
REF: 40-p. 280

711. The Australia antigen, discovered in 1963 by Blumberg, is also known as the antigen of
A. hepatitis A
B. hepatitis B
C. hepatitis C
D. hepatitis D
REF: 40-p. 273

712. The form of hepatitis which is spread by contaminated blood or blood products is termed
A. hepatitis A
B. hepatitis B
C. hepatitis C
D. hepatitis D
REF: 40-p. 280

713. The form of hepatitis which is transmitted by the oral-fecal route is termed
A. hepatitis A
B. hepatitis B
C. hepatitis C
D. hepatitis D
REF: 40-p. 277

714. The detection of the presence of anti-HAV by RIA in a patient's serum sample is indicative of
A. hepatitis A
B. hepatitis B
C. hepatitis C
D. hepatitis D
REF: 40-p. 277

715. Advantages of the RIA technique for hepatitis-associated antigens (HAA) over conventional methods such as CEP, AGD, and CF include all of the following EXCEPT
A. RIA is more sensitive
B. RIA provides quantitative data
C. RIA is simpler to perform
D. RIA uses labeled antiserum instead of antigen
REF: 36-p. 314

716. Total serum concentrations of T_3 may be low in patients with all of the following conditions EXCEPT
A. neonatal status
B. elderly status
C. hepatic disease
D. fasting state
REF: 40-p. 248

717. The metabolically inert iodothyronine which corresponds reciprocally to the concentration of metabolically active T_3 and is useful in elucidating peripheral metabolism of thyroid hormones is known as

A. tetraiodothyroacetic acid (tetrac)
B. reverse triiodothyronine (rT_3)
C. reverse tetraiodothyronine (rT_4)
D. pre-pro T_3
REF: 40-p. 251

718. The purpose of the addition of ANS (8 anilino naphthlenesulfonic acid) in some RIA tests for T4 is to

A. inhibit the binding of T4 to the endogenous binding proteins (TBG, TBPA, and albumin)
B. enhance the binding of T4 to the endogenous binding proteins (TBG, TBPA, and albumin)
C. extract the T4 from serum TBG binding, thus enabling the measurement of free T4
D. extract the T3 from serum TBG binding, thus eliminating interference
REF: 40-p. 249

719. T_3 by RIA is most helpful in the diagnosis of

A. hypothyroidism
B. hyperthyroidism
C. thyroiditis
D. thyroid carcinoma
REF: 32-p. 468

720. The greatest clinical utility of measuring TSH by RIA is in differentiating

A. primary from secondary hypothyroidism
B. Graves' from Plummer's disease
C. Hashimoto's thyroiditis from Reidel's struma
D. thyroid adenoma from cyst
REF: 32-p. 468

721. Serum TSH levels are generally ____________ in hypothyroidism and ____________ in hyperthyroidism.

A. decreased; elevated
B. decreased; normal
C. normal; elevated
D. elevated; decreased
REF: 36-p. 312

722. In the TSH RIA procedure, high concentrations of which of the following hormones are likely to cross-react with the TSH molecule?
A. T_3
B. HCG
C. PTH
D. TBG
REF: 36-p. 312

723. TSH by RIA is a valuable diagnostic tool in differentiating
A. Graves' from Plummer's disease
B. primary from secondary hypothyroidism
C. thyroid adenoma from cyst
D. thyroid carcinoma from cyst
REF: 36-p. 312

724. Calcitonin, a hormone involved in calcium metabolism, is produced in the
A. parathyroid glands
B. thyroid gland
C. pancreas
D. anterior pituitary
REF: 32-p. 241

725. An important clinical application of measurement of calcitonin levels by RIA is in the diagnosis of
A. hyperparathyroidism
B. medullary carcinoma of the thyroid
C. Hashimoto's thyroiditis
D. parathyroid adenoma
REF: 40-p. 236

726. A person with clinical features of acromegaly is likely to be tested for which hormonal aberration?
A. Elevated TSH levels
B. Depressed TSH levels
C. Elevated HGH levels
D. Depressed HGH levels
REF: 40-p. 208

727. PTH, or parathormone, which is produced by the parathyroid glands, is important in the regulation of
A. iodine
B. calcium
C. tyrosine
D. thyrotropin
REF: 32-p. 256

728. Hypercalcemia, in conjunction with elevated levels of circulating PTH, is indicative of which disease process?
A. Hypoparathyroidism
B. Hyperparathyroidism
C. Hypothyroidism
D. Hyperthyroidism
REF: 40-p. 230

729. Serum specimens drawn for PTH by RIA require all of the following conditions EXCEPT
A. they should be frozen promptly after collection
B. they should be collected in the early a.m.
C. they should be collected postprandially
D. they should be collected in the fasting state
REF: 40-p. 228

730. The greatest clinical utility in the measurement of circulating levels of PTH by RIA has been in the diagnosis of
A. hypothyroidism
B. hypoparathyroidism
C. hyperthyroidism
D. hyperparathyroidism
REF: 40-p. 230

731. The effect of the hormone gastrin, secreted by the gastric antrum, is to
A. stimulate gastric acid secretion
B. suppress gastric acid secretion
C. increase gastric motility
D. decrease gastric motility
REF: 40-p. 291

732. Collection of serum samples for gastrin RIA requires that the patient
A. is in a 20-minute postprandial state
B. is in a fasting state overnight
C. have an N-G tube in place
D. be premedicated with a vagal stimulator
REF: 40-p. 293

733. The most common cause of inappropriate hypergastrinemia is the presence of a gastrinoma, also known as
A. Addison's disease
B. Zollinger-Ellison syndrome
C. Cushing's syndrome
D. G-cell hyperplasia
REF: 40-p. 294

734. Serum gastrin levels are of diagnostic significance in evaluating
A. duodenal from peptic ulcer disease
B. Zollinger-Ellison syndrome from pernicious anemia
C. blind loop syndrome from malabsorption
D. esophageal reflux syndrome from gastric carcinoma
REF: 36-p. 313

735. In collection of a serum sample from a patient for bile acid assay, the patient should be
A. in a 90-minute postprandial state
B. in a 12-hour fasting state
C. in a supine position
D. in an upright position
REF: 40-p. 304

736. Interpretation of the postprandial serum bile-acid test should be made in light of knowledge about the condition of the patient's
A. duodenal loop
B. jejunum
C. terminal ileum
D. gastric antrum
REF: 40-p. 304

737. Serum bile acid assay has found clinical usefulness in all of the following areas EXCEPT
A. evaluating the progress of patients with documented hepatitis
B. differentiating the various types of liver disease
C. early evaluation of drug-induced liver disease
D. as an aid in the treatment of alcoholic liver disease
REF: 40-p. 305

738. Order the following routes of drug administration methods in the sequence of fastest to slowest rate of peak concentration in the circulation.
A. Intramuscular, intravenous, oral
B. Oral, intravenous, intramuscular
C. Oral, intravenous, intramuscular
D. Intravenous, intramuscular, oral
REF: 32-p. 469

739. The two *major* routes of drug removal from the circulation are the following.
A. Renal and fecal removal
B. Renal and hepatic removal
C. Fecal and hepatic removal
D. Renal and sweat glands removal
REF: 32-p. 470

740. In general, the therapeutic range or window for digoxin, the digitalis glycoside which controls cardiac arrythmias, is
A. 0-1.0 pg/ml
B. 1.0 to 2.1 pg/ml
C. 0-1.0 ng/ml
D. 1.0-2.1 ng/ml
REF: 32-p. 470

741. The standard time when blood for digoxin concentration measurements should be drawn is approximately ____________ hours after the last digoxin dose was taken.
A. 2
B. 4
C. 6
D. 8
REF: 32-p. 470

742. Serum digoxin concentrations may be affected by all the following conditions EXCEPT the
A. absorption ability of the patient
B. volume of distribution in the patient
C. fecal excretion of digoxin
D. urinary excretion of digoxin
REF: 40-p. 315

743. A toxic level of digoxin determined from a serum digoxin radioassay is not definitive for digoxin intoxication. What other factors govern the effectiveness of digitalis?
A. Renal function of the patient
B. Thyroid status of the patient
C. Hepatic disorder of the patient
D. All of the above
E. A and B only
F. A and C only
REF: 36-p. 307

744. In general, the therapeutic range for digitoxin, another digitalis glycoside structurally similar to digoxin, is
A. 1.0–2.6 pg/ml
B. 10–26 pg/ml
C. 1.0–2.6 ng/ml
D. 10–26 ng/ml
REF: 32-p. 470

745. A CK-B (creatinine-kinase-B isoenzyme) serum level taken on a patient 2 days after a myocardial infarct will be
A. elevated
B. diminished
C. normal
D. absent
REF: 40-p. 329

746. Serum samples for measurement of CK-B (creatinine-kinase-B isoenzyme) by RIA on patients with acute myocardial infarction should be obtained within approximately ____________ hours after insult.
A. 0-6
B. 6-12
C. 12-24
D. 24-36
REF: 40-pp. 329-330

747. The serum level of CK-B (creatinine-kinase-B isoenzyme), in addition to being elevated in cases of acute myocardial infarction, is also elevated in
A. chronic liver disease
B. acute CVA
C. ischemic heart disease
D. digoxin toxicity
REF: 40-p. 330

748. The low molecular weight protein which is found only in skeletal and cardiac striated muscle and which is elevated in patients post myocardial infarction is known as
A. myoglobin
B. calcitonin
C. lactoferrin
D. myosin
REF: 40-p. 330

749. Samples for a serum myoglobin assay by RIA must be obtained within ____________ hours after the onset of symptoms.
A. 0-4
B. 4-8
C. 8-12
D. 12-24
REF: 40-p. 332

750. Falsely low levels of vitamin B_{12} by radioassay can occur as a result of prior administration of ____________ to the patient.

A. biotin
B. riboflavin
C. folic acid
D. ascorbic acid
REF: 40-p. 338

751. Vitamin B_{12} levels less than 200 pg/ml by RIA are most likely indicative of which of the following disorders?

A. Pernicious anemia
B. Malabsorption syndrome
C. Acute renal failure
D. All of the above
E. A and B only
REF: 36-p. 317

752. The normal circulating level of vitamin B-12 is approximately

A. 10-30 ng/ml
B. 150-300 ng/ml
C. 130-700 pg/ml
D. 900-1500 pg/ml
REF: 32-p. 474

753. The disease entity which is caused by long-term vitamin B-12 deficiency is called

A. microcytic anemia
B. sickle cell anemia
C. megaloblastic anemia
D. aplastic anemia
REF: 32-p. 474

754. The specific reactor substance used in vitamin B-12 RIA procedures is

A. transcobalamin I
B. transcobalamin II
C. folic acid
D. hog intrinsic factor
REF: 32-p. 475

755. The radiolabel used in vitamin B-12 radioimmunoassay methods is
A. ^{125}I
B. ^{75}Se
C. ^{57}Co
D. ^{131}I
REF: 32-p. 475

756. In the folate radioassay, the specific folate reactor substance or binder is generally obtained from
A. hog's intestine
B. cow's milk
C. cow's rumen
D. hog's stomach
REF: 32-p. 475

757. Special precautions which should be taken when dealing with samples for folate analysis include
A. protection from heat
B. protection from light
C. addition of ascorbic acid
D. all of the above
E. A and B only
REF: 32-p. 475

758. Factors which influence the values determined for insulin levels by RIA include all of the following EXCEPT
A. hemolysis of the sample
B. nonfrozen samples
C. prior insulin therapy of patient
D. incomplete urine collection
REF: 36-p. 313

759. The subunit which is immunologically identical for the glycoprotein hormones FSH, LH, TSH, and HCG is the
A. alpha subunit
B. beta subunit
C. gamma subunit
D. delta subunit
REF: 34-p. 43

760. Estriol, the most abundant of the estrogens produced and secreted by the feto-placental unit, shows increased levels in which of the following conditions?

A. Fetal death
B. Normal pregnancy
C. Preeclampsia
D. Molar pregnancy
REF: 36-p. 316

761. HCG levels determined by RIA methods has its greatest clinical utility in diagnosing

A. fetal death
B. fetal distress
C. early pregnancy
D. preeclampsia
REF: 36-p. 317

762. The measurement of AFP (alpha-fetoprotein) by RIA is useful in the diagnosis of

A. fetal developmental defects
B. hepatoblastoma
C. teratocarcinoma of the ovaries
D. liver metastases
E. all of the above
F. A and C only
REF: 40-p. 410

763. The most important diagnostic test for gestational trophoblastic diseases, such as hydatidiform mole or choriocarcinoma, is the measurement of

A. AFP
B. CEA
C. HCG
D. LH
REF: 40-p. 411

764. Levels of CEA (carcinoembryonic antigen) above 2.5 ng/ml in noncancerous conditions may be caused by all of the following EXCEPT

A. smoking
B. advanced age
C. benign breast disease
D. gastrointestinal disease
REF: 40-p. 408

765. CEA levels are generally of no aid in differentiation of
- **A.** benign from malignant breast disease
- **B.** benign from malignant lung disease
- **C.** benign from malignant colon disease
- **D.** benign from malignant hepatic disease

REF: 40-p. 409

766. The hormonal negative feedback system which regulates sodium and potassium balance, and ultimately blood pressure, is known as the
- **A.** renin-aldosterone-angiotensin axis
- **B.** ADH-aldosterone-angiotensin axis
- **C.** renin-angiotensin-aldosterone axis
- **D.** aldosterone-ADH-renin axis

REF: 40-p. 435

767. When collecting blood samples for RIA plasma renin levels, it is important that the patient
- **A.** ambulate for at least 1 hour prior to sample collection
- **B.** recline for at least 1 hour prior to sample collection
- **C.** eat a high sodium diet for 5 days prior to collection of sample
- **D.** restrict his/her diet to moderate levels of sodium for 5 days prior to collection of sample
- **E.** A and C only
- **F.** B and C only
- **G.** A and D only

REF: 40-p. 436

768. When estimating plasma renin levels using RIA, angiotensin I is first generated in the sample by altering the
- **A.** temperature
- **B.** pH
- **C.** osmolality
- **D.** titer

REF: 36-p. 309

769. When blood is being collected for a renin level, what special precaution(s) must be observed?
- **A.** Sample must be collected in an EDTA-coated tube
- **B.** Sample must be separated in a refrigerated centrifuge
- **C.** Sample should be placed on ice until assayed
- **D.** All of the above

REF: 40-p. 437

770. When performing plasma renin level assays, which of the following substances is(are) actually measured?
- **A.** Renin
- **B.** Angiotensin I
- **C.** Angiotensin II
- **D.** Aldosterone
- **E.** A and B
- **F.** B and C

REF: 40-p. 437

771. Plasma renin activity measurements are clinically useful in differentiating the various forms of
- **A.** hypertension
- **B.** arteriosclerotic disease
- **C.** carcinoma
- **D.** renal disease

REF: 40-p. 443

772. Gentamicin, which may be measured radioimmunologically, belongs to the class of drugs known as
- **A.** anticonvulsants
- **B.** bronchodilators
- **C.** antibiotics
- **D.** vasodilators

REF: 40-p. 401

773. All of the following may be measured by RIA methods EXCEPT
- **A.** steroid hormones
- **B.** blood volume
- **C.** chemotherapeutic drugs
- **D.** tumor markers

REF: 38-p. 326

774. In quality control procedures, the smaller the standard deviation measured in a series of measurement, the higher the assay's
A. sensitivity
B. specificity
C. accuracy
D. precision
REF: 32-p. 460

775. The degree of agreement between duplicate or triplicate measurements of the same sample can be determined using which of the following statistical measures?
A. Mean
B. Standard deviation
C. Coefficient of variation
D. Correlation coefficient
REF: 34-p. 284

776. The optimum number of quality control samples which should be run with each assay is
A. 1
B. 2
C. 3
D. 4
REF: 34-p. 285

777. The chart which is used to plot daily control values and which allows the technologist to determine runs of unacceptable standards is called a
A. Dickson chart
B. Scatchard plot
C. Levey-Jennings chart
D. Chi-square plot
REF: 34-p. 286

778. Long-term monitoring of an assay's performance using the quality control reference samples can be accomplished utilizing which of the following methods?
A. Time windows
B. Trigg's technique
C. CUSUM technique
D. All of the above
E. B and C only
REF: 34-p. 290

779. The shape of the standard curve of a particular assay may change with time, and can be a serious problem in certain situations. This change in shape may be due to all of the following EXCEPT

A. changes in antibody lots
B. incubation time
C. incubation temperature
D. uniform deterioration of standards

REF: 34-p. 296

12. THYROID GLAND

DIRECTIONS: Each of the questions or incomplete statements below is followed by a list of suggested answers or completions. Select the **one** that is **BEST** in each case.

---

780. The thyroid gland is
- **A.** an exocrine gland
- **B.** an apocrine gland
- **C.** an endocrine gland
- **D.** an adenine gland

REF: 1-p. 384

781. In the human fetus, the thyroid becomes functional
- **A.** during the third month of gestation
- **B.** during the sixth month of gestation
- **C.** during the ninth month of gestation
- **D.** at birth

REF: 1-p. 384

782. As a result of its embryonic migration, thyroid tissue may be found from
A. the suprasternal notch to the level of T12
B. the base of the tongue to the level of the diaphragm
C. the level of the diaphragm to L-5
D. the thyroid cartilage to the suprasternal notch exclusively
REF: 1-p. 384

783. Other structures associated with the thyroid gland, in addition to its two relatively symmetrical lobes, include which of the following?
A. A pyramidal lobe
B. An isthmus
C. Parathyroid glands
D. All of the above
E. A and C only
REF: 32-p. 241

784. The thyroid extracts two substances from the blood for use in hormonogenesis. These are ____________ and ____________.
A. iodine; thyroglobulin
B. iodine; thyrobinding globulin
C. iodide; tyrosine
D. iodine; thyroxine
REF: 40-p. 246

785. The function of the thyroid's cuboidal epithelial cells is to
A. store hormone
B. synthesize hormone
C. trap iodide from the blood
D. all of the above
E. B and C only
REF: 1-p. 385

786. After radioiodide is ingested by the patient, what is its thyroidal metabolic pathway?

A. Gut absorption, plasma, body tissues, protein binding in circulation, thyroidal trapping, thyroidal organification, thyroidal secretion, blood stream

B. Gut absorption, plasma, thyroidal trapping, thyroidal organification, thyroidal secretion, protein binding in circulation, body tissues

C. Gut absorption, protein binding in circulation, thyroidal trapping, thyroidal organification, thyroidal secretion, body tissues

REF: 1-p. 387

787. The amino acid extracted by the thyroid gland to be used in the synthesis of hormones is

A. thyronine

B. thyroglobulin

C. thyroxine

D. tyrosine

REF: 34-p. 378

788. The hormones which the thyroid gland produces include all of the following EXCEPT

A. calcitonin

B. thyroxine

C. triiodothyronine

D. TSH

REF: 32-p. 241

789. After synthesis, the thyroid hormones T3 and T4 are stored in the ____________ until needed for use in the body.

A. cuboidal epithelium of the thyroid

B. parathyroid glands

C. adenohypophysis

D. colloidal thyroid follicles

REF: 33-p. 104

790. Hormone is stored in the thyroid gland in the form of
A. triiodothyronine
B. thyrotropin
C. thyroxine
D. all of the above
E. A and C only
REF: 1-p. 387

791. Thyroid hormone, once it has been synthesized in the follicle, is stored in the form of a large protein molecule, ___________, until needed by the body.
A. monoiodotyrosine
B. diiodotyrosine
C. thyroxine
D. thyroglobulin
REF: 1-p. 387

792. The thyroid hormone which is in the greatest abundance in the bloodstream is
A. triiodothyronine
B. thyroxine
C. calcitonin
D. TSH
REF: 33-p. 104; 33-p. 241

793. The more metabolically active of the thyroid hormones T3 and T4 is
A. triiodothyronine
B. thyroxine
REF: 33-p. 104; 33-p. 241

794. The bulk of circulating thyroid hormone is
A. free, unbound
B. TBG bound
C. TBPA bound
D. albumin bound
REF: 33-p. 104

795. Most of the circulating thyroid hormone is bound to ___________ in the blood.
A. erythrocytes
B. plasma proteins
C. transferrin
D. leukocytes
REF: 32-p. 242

796. Calcitonin, the blood calcium-regulating polypeptide hormone manufactured by the thyroid, is secreted by the
A. parafollicular cells
B. C cells
C. cuboidal epithelial
D. all of the above
E. A and B only
REF: 32-p. 241

797. The hypothalamic pituitary thyroid axis is defined as the relationship between
A. ACTH, TRH, and TSH
B. TRH, TSH, and thyroxine
C. T3 and T4
D. ADH, TRH, and T4
REF: 1-p. 384

798. The negative feedback mechanism, which controls the activities of the thyroid gland, is regulated by the amount of ____________ thyroid hormone in the blood.
A. free
B. protein-bound
C. denatured
D. normalized
REF: 40-p. 251

799. The thyroid gland is under the *direct* control of
A. the posterior pituitary
B. the anterior pituitary
C. the parathyroid glands
D. the hypothalamus
REF: 1-p. 384

800. TSH, or thyroid stimulating hormone, is secreted by the
A. hypothalamus
B. pituitary gland
C. parathyroid glands
D. thyroid gland
REF: 1-p. 384

801. Direct actions of TSH include all of the following EXCEPT

A. stimulates thyroid cell growth
B. increases iodide incorporation
C. increases bodily metabolism
D. stimulates hormone release from the thyroid
REF: 36-p. 235

802. The hormone which stimulates the release of TSH from the anterior pituitary is

A. ACTH
B. TRH
C. T3
D. T4
REF: 1-p. 384

803. The element which is essential for normal thyroid function is

A. iron
B. iodine
C. chlorine
D. fluorine
REF: 32-p. 241

804. Isotopes of iodine which have been used in evaluating thyroid function include all of the following EXCEPT

A. ^{127}I
B. ^{123}I
C. ^{131}I
D. ^{132}I
REF: 32-p. 246

805. Euthyroidism refers to the condition of the thyroid as being

A. overactive
B. normal
C. underactive
D. oversecreting
REF: 17-p. 268

806. Hypothyroidism may be caused by all of the following EXCEPT
A. iodine deficiency
B. inherited enzyme deficiency
C. post radioiodine ablation
D. end stage toxic goiter
E. none of the above
REF: 41-p. 846

807. The condition known as myxedema is the end stage of
A. hyperthyroidism
B. hypothyroidism
C. Graves' disease
D. Plummer's disease
REF: 1-p. 399

808. Which of the following conditions occurs as a result of thyroid deficiency in infancy?
A. Down's syndrome
B. Mongolism
C. Cretinism
D. Myxedema
REF: 1-p. 399

809. Pre-tibial myxedema is a common characteristic of patients with
A. primary hypothyroidism
B. secondary hypothyroidism
C. tertiary hypothyroidism
D. Graves' disease
REF: 1-p. 397

810. Primary hypothyroidism is due to
A. failure of the pituitary to secrete TSH
B. failure of the hypothalamus to secrete TSH
C. failure of the gland itself
D. all of the above
REF: 41-p. 843

811. Secondary hypothyroidism is due to
A. failure of the pituitary to secrete TSH
B. failure of the hypothalamus to secrete TRH
C. failure of the gland itself
D. none of the above
REF: 41-p. 843

812. Hashimoto's thyroiditis is also known as
A. acute suppurative thyroiditis
B. subacute thyroiditis
C. nonsuppurative thyroiditis
D. chronic lymphocytic thyroiditis
REF: 41-p. 995

813. Which of the following conditions is characterized by hypermetabolism with a nodular gland?
A. Graves' disease
B. Hashimoto's thyroiditis
C. Myxedema
D. Plummer's disease
REF: 1-p. 397

814. Plummer's disease is another name for
A. toxic diffuse goiter
B. toxic nodular goiter
C. hypothyroid goiter
D. Graves' disease
REF: 1-p. 398

815. Exophthalmos is a common characteristic of which condition(s)?
A. Hyperthyroidism
B. Thyrotoxicosis
C. Graves' disease
D. All of the above
E. A and C only
REF: 1-p. 397

816. Graves' disease may be distinguished from Plummer's disease by
A. the presence of circulating LATS
B. the absence of a hypermetabolic state
C. an elevated TSH level
D. all of the above
E. A and C only
REF: 1-p. 398

817. Treatments for hyperthyroidism include all of the following EXCEPT
A. thyroidectomy
B. antithyroid medications
C. ^{131}I therapy
D. TSH therapy
REF: 41-p. 814; 38-p. 109

818. Hyperthyroidism caused by excessive self-administration of exogenous thyroid extract is referred to as
A. Graves' disease
B. Plummer's disease
C. Hashimoto's thyrotoxicosis
D. thyrotoxicosis factitia
REF: 41-p. 598

819. In the radioiodine thyroid uptake procedure
A. the amount of fecal excretion reflects the functional level of the gland
B. the amount localized in the thyroid gland reflects the functional status of the gland
C. the amount absorbed by the gastric mucosa reflects the functional status of the gland
D. the amount ingested reflects the functional status of the gland
REF: 38-p. 330

820. The mechanism of localization used by the thyroid in trapping iodide ions is
A. phagocytosis
B. ion exchange
C. active transport
D. compartmental localization
REF: 41-p. 34

821. Indications for performing a radioiodine uptake study include all of the following except
A. suspicion of hyperthyroidism
B. suspicion of hypothyroidism
C. suspicion of a thyroid cyst
D. suspicion of pituitary failure
REF: 36-p. 250

822. The major use of the radioiodine thyroid uptake test is in distinguishing
A. hypofunction from normal function
B. hyperfunction from normal function
C. hyperfunction from hypofunction
D. Graves' from Plummer's disease
REF: 38-p. 336

823. Patient preparation for radioiodine administration for a thyroid uptake include
A. 10 drops of SSKI the day before
B. NPO for 12 hours
C. $KClO_4$ 30 minutes after
D. Lugol's solution 3 days before and 3 days after
REF: 36-p. 251

824. The radiopharmaceutical of choice for performing a pediatric uptake is
A. ^{127}I sodium iodide
B. ^{131}I sodium iodide
C. ^{123}I sodium iodide
D. ^{99m}Tc pertechnetate
REF: 32-p. 249

825. The usual route of administration of radioiodine for a thyroid uptake test is
A. intravenous
B. oral
C. intramuscular
D. intrathyroidal
REF: 36-p. 251

826. The standard equation for determination of a thyroid uptake is

A. $\frac{\text{(standard cpm - thigh cpm)}}{\text{neck cpm}} \times 100$

B. $\frac{\text{(standard cpm - neck cpm)}}{\text{thigh cpm}} \times 100$

C. $\frac{\text{(neck cpm - thigh cpm)}}{\text{standard cpm}} \times 100$

D. $\frac{\text{(standard cpm - neck cpm)}}{\text{standard cpm}} \times 100$

REF: 36-p. 251

827. The normal values for a radioactive iodine uptake test have generally
A. increased over the years
B. decreased over the years
C. remained stable over the years
REF: 36-p. 250

828. The average normal range for a 2-hour uptake using radioiodine is
A. 0.5-8.9%
B. 10.1-15.6%
C. 20.5-30.5%
D. 30.7-40.2%
REF: 36-p. 255

829. The average normal range for a 24-hour uptake using radioiodine is
A. 2-10%
B. 10-30%
C. 30-40%
D. 40-50%
REF: 36-p. 251

830. An early 2-6 hours thyroid uptake measurement may be crucial in making a diagnosis of
A. primary hypothyroidism
B. Hashimoto's thyroiditis
C. Graves' disease
D. nonfunctioning nodule
REF: 36-p. 251

831. Elevated radioiodine uptake measurements can be seen in
A. acute renal failure
B. iodine deficiency
C. Hashimoto's thyroiditis
D. all of the above
E. A and B only
REF: 32-p. 248

832. The following condition(s) decrease(s) uptake of radioiodine by the thyroid.
A. Edema
B. Iodine deficiency
C. Renal failure
D. Chronic liver disease
E. All of the above
F. A and C only
REF: 32-p. 248

833. All of the following commonly used pharmaceuticals may decrease the radioiodine uptake EXCEPT
A. cough mixtures and expectorants
B. tincture of iodine
C. vaginal suppositories
D. vitamin C
REF: 32-p. 247

834. If the extrathyroidal iodine pool is increased, the percent radioiodine uptake will be
A. decreased
B. increased
C. unchanged
REF: 38-p. 331

835. The physical half-life and primary energy peak of ^{123}I are
A. 8.06 days; 364 keV
B. 60 days; 35 keV
C. 6 hours; 140 keV
D. 13.6 hours; 159 keV
REF: 36-p. 456

836. Advantages of using ^{123}I over ^{131}I in performing thyroid studies include all of the following EXCEPT

A. it is less costly
B. it gives a significantly lesser radiation dose to the patient
C. it emits an energy more suited to gamma camera imaging
D. all of the above
E. B and C only
REF: 1-p. 391

837. The purpose of a thyroid uptake study is

A. to study the rate of accumulation, incorporation, and release of radioiodine
B. to assess pituitary integrity
C. to indirectly study thyroid physiology
D. all of the above
E. A and C only
REF: 36-p. 250

838. The number of images usually taken for a ^{131}I thyroid uptake is

A. two
B. four
C. six
D. none
REF: 36-p. 251

839. The TSH stimulation study is used to measure

A. trapping ability of the thyroid
B. organification ability of the thyroid
C. thyroid reserve
D. thyroid hormones
REF: 38-p. 336

840. The TSH stimulation test is helpful in differentiating

A. Graves' disease from Plummer's disease
B. primary from secondary hypothyroidism
C. primary from secondary hyperthyroidism
D. primary from secondary hypoparathyroidism
REF: 36-p. 239

841. An abnormal response (no substantial increase in uptake) on a TSH stimulation test is seen in all of the following conditions EXCEPT
A. nontoxic multinodular goiter
B. Hashimoto's thyroiditis
C. post ^{131}I therapy for Graves' disease
D. hypopituitarism
REF: 38-p. 336

842. A patient whose baseline uptake was 2% (hypothyroid by this lab), and whose uptake increased to 10% after TSH stimulation, probably has
A. a normal gland
B. hypopituitarism
C. secondary hypothyroidism
D. all of the above
E. B and C only
REF: 38-p. 336

843. The rationale of the thyroid suppression test rests on the concept of the normal hypothalamic pituitary thyroid axis. With this in mind, administration of exogenous T3 should
A. suppress pituitary TSH release
B. stimulate hypothalamic TRH release
C. diminish normal thyroid function
D. all of the above
E. A and C only
REF: 33-p. 116

844. The thyroid suppression test may be performed using
A. Cytomel
B. triiodothyronine
C. thyroxine
D. all of the above
E. A and B only
REF: 33-p. 116

845. When used in conjunction with the radioiodine thyroid uptake, the Cytomel suppression test demonstrates that failure of the baseline radioiodine uptake to be suppressed by more than ____________ is evidence of autonomy.
A. 20%
B. 30%
C. 40%
D. 50%
REF: 38-p. 336

846. In a Cytomel suppression study, the second study usually follows the first by
A. 2 hours
B. 2 days
C. 3 days
D. 5 days
REF: 36-p. 242

847. Performing a thyroid scan in conjunction with a T3 suppression test is helpful in cases of
A. hot nodules
B. hypofunction
C. cold nodules
D. Plummer's disease
E. A and D only
REF: 1-p. 406

848. In the Cytomel suppression test, the radioiodine uptake in a patient with hyperthyroidism will
A. decrease
B. increase
C. remain the same
REF: 38-p. 336

849. TRH (thyrotropin-releasing hormone) stimulation tests are used to
A. determine pituitary integrity
B. differentiate secondary from tertiary hypothyroidism
C. differentiate primary from secondary hyperthyroidism
D. all of the above
E. A and B only
REF: 38-p. 337

850. In normal subjects, intravenous administration of TRH would be followed by
A. a prompt decrease in serum TSH levels
B. a prompt increase in serum TSH levels
C. a gradual rise of serum TSH levels over 3 days
D. a gradual decline of serum TSH levels over 3 days
REF: 41-p. 367

851. The TRH stimulation test may, in the future, replace the Cytomel suppression test because
A. repeated uptakes are not necessary, so problems with time and background are eliminated
B. TRH has no adverse side effects on the patients, whereas Cytomel does
C. TRH stimulation is simpler, cheaper, and faster than the T3 suppression test
D. all of the above
E. A and C only
REF: 41-p. 372

852. The iodide-washout test is used to study patients with a suspected
A. trapping defect
B. organification defect
C. synthesis defect
D. secretion defect
REF: 36-p. 246

853. Diseases which typically demonstrate a positive perchlorate washout study include
A. Graves' disease
B. Hashimoto's thyroditis
C. thyroid carcinoma
D. all of the above
E. B and C only
REF: 36-p. 246

854. In the perchlorate discharge test, a decrease in the baseline uptake of ____________ or more indicates an organification defect.

A. 10%
B. 40%
C. 60%
D. 75%
REF: 38-p. 336

855. A patient with a borderline high radioiodine uptake may be misdiagnosed as hyperthyroid. Which of the following tests would be helpful in differentiating whether the patient is truly hyperthyroid or merely a high normal?

A. TSH stimulation test
B. Perchlorate discharge test
C. Cytomel suppression test
D. TRH stimulation test
REF: 33-p. 116

856. All of the following procedures require the use of multiple radioiodine uptake determinations EXCEPT

A. perchlorate washout test
B. TSH stimulation test
C. Cytomel suppression test
D. TRH stimulation test
REF: 36-p. 248

857. The following procedure(s) can be started and completed in one day.

A. Perchlorate washout study
B. Thyroid suppression study
C. TSH stimulation study
D. TRH stimulation study
E. All of the above
F. A and D only
REF: 36-p. 246

858. Radioiodine, which is used for thyroid uptakes, is usually administered ____________, while pertechnetate, for scanning purposes, is given ____________.
A. orally; orally
B. intravenously; orally
C. intravenously; intravenously
D. orally; intravenously
REF: 36-p. 251

859. The most common radionuclides used to scan the thyroid gland include all of the following EXCEPT
A. ^{131}I sodium iodide
B. ^{123}I sodium iodide
C. ^{99m}Tc sodium pertechnetate
D. ^{125}I sodium iodide
REF: 1-p. 401

860. The purpose of a thyroid scan is to elucidate information regarding
A. size, shape, and position of the gland
B. function of the gland
C. nodularity of the gland
D. all of the above
E. A and C only
REF: 1-p. 400

861. The anatomical landmarks most commonly used in thyroid scintigraphy are
A. the cricoid cartilage and the suprasternal notch
B. the suprasternal notch and the xiphoid process
C. the thyroid cartilage and the suprasternal notch
D. the Adam's apple and the suprasternal notch
E. A and C only
F. C and D only
REF: 36-p. 446

862. An image taken of a normal thyroid gland may demonstrate all of the following EXCEPT
A. the presence of a pyramidal lobe
B. the right lobe larger than the left
C. heterogenous distribution of activity
D. decreased activity in the isthmus
REF: 17-p. 266

863. Maximum uptake of $^{99m}TcO_4^-$ by the thyroid gland takes place approximately ____________ after intravenous injection.
A. 24 hours
B. 6 hours
C. 2 minutes
D. 20 minutes
REF: 33-p. 116

864. When using ^{99m}Tc sodium pertechnetate as a thyroid imaging agent, which function(s) of the thyroid gland is (are) imaged?
A. Trapping ability
B. Organification ability
C. Trapping and organification ability
D. Synthesizing ability
REF: 41-p. 285; 32-p. 65

865. Thyroidal trapping of ^{99m}Tc-sodium pertechnetate is inhibited by
A. perchlorate
B. methimazole
C. thiocyanate
D. propylthiouracil
E. all of the above
F. A and C only
REF: 41-p. 287; 34-p. 115

866. Patient preparation for a ^{99m}Tc pertechnetate thyroid scan consists of
A. a 12-hour fast
B. nothing
C. 0.5 cc of KCl given IV
D. 10 drops of Lugol's solution
REF: 36-p. 445

867. In scanning the thyroid using ^{131}I or ^{123}I sodium iodide, the optimal interval between radiopharmaceutical administration and scanning is
A. 20 minutes
B. 4 hours
C. 6 hours
D. 24 hours
REF: 36-p. 447

868. Radionuclides which have been used to image the thyroid gland include all of the following EXCEPT
A. Thallium-201
B. Iodine-131
C. Technetium-99m
D. Xenon-133
REF: 38-p. 330

869. The appearance of both "hot" and "cold" nodules in a euthyroid gland is usually indicative of
A. multinodular goiter
B. Hashimoto's thyroiditis
C. Graves' disease
D. carcinoma
REF: 17-p. 270

870. A solitary "cold" nodule found in an otherwise normal thyroid gland is indicative of a ____________ in approximately 25% of the cases.
A. cyst
B. thyrotoxic goiter
C. toxic adenoma
D. carcinoma
REF: 1-p. 403

871. The differential diagnosis of a "cold" nodule seen on conventional thyroid scintigraphy includes all of the following conditions EXCEPT
A. thyroid cyst
B. hemorrhage
C. localized thyroiditis
D. hyperplastic adenoma
REF: 41-p. 306

872. Which of the following diagnostic modalities is usually used after demonstration of a solitary "cold" nodule is seen on thyroid scintigraphy?
A. Ultrasonography
B. Computerized tomography
C. Biopsy
D. Contrast angiography
REF: 41-p. 306

873. If a patient who has a solitary nodule on palpation has a normal ^{99m}Tc pertechnetate thyroid scan, what would be the next step?
A. Surgery to remove the nodule
B. Cytomel suppression test
C. Perchlorate discharge study
D. ^{123}I sodium iodide scan
REF: 1-p. 402

874. The radiopharmaceutical of choice for imaging a substernal thyroid is
A. ^{125}I sodium iodide
B. ^{99m}Tc pertechnetate
C. ^{131}I sodium iodide
D. ^{67}Ga citrate
REF: 37-p. 104

875. A useful application of thyroid scintigraphy is in locating functioning ectopic thyroid tissue, which can be found in which of the following anatomical areas?
A. Sublingual
B. Retrosternal
C. Orbital
D. All of the above
E. A and B only
REF: 41-p. 310

876. When imaging with both ^{99m}Tc pertechnetate and radioiodine fails in the case of Hashimoto's thyroiditis, which of the following radiopharmaceuticals may be used as an alternative?
A. Thallium-201
B. Selenomethionine-75
C. Gallium-67
D. All of the above
E. B and C only
REF: 41-p. 309

877. A patient with a hot nodule on a ^{99m}Tc pertechnetate scan is referred back to the Nuclear Medicine department for determination of the nodule's autonomy. The best test to determine this would be
A. TSH stimulation test
B. TRH stimulation test
C. Cytomel suppression test
D. Perchlorate discharge study
REF: 38-p. 336

878. Which of the following radiopharmaceuticals allows assessment of the trapping ability of the thyroid, but no organification information?
A. ^{131}I sodium iodide
B. ^{99m}Tc pertechnetate
C. ^{123}I sodium iodide
D. ^{75}Se selenomethionine
REF: 32-p. 249

879. The most commonly used radionuclide utilized in in vitro thyroid determinations is
A. ^{123}I
B. ^{125}I
C. ^{127}I
D. ^{131}I
REF: 32-p. 452

880. The in vitro T3 uptake test is
A. a direct measure of T3
B. an indirect measure of T4
C. an indirect measure of TBG
D. an indirect measure of T3
E. A and C only
F. B and C only
REF: 33-p. 110

881. Which of the following plasma carrier proteins determine the general binding patterns for the thyroid hormones and therefore is the determining factor in the utility of the T3 uptake and T4 tests?
A. Thyroglobulin
B. Albumin
C. TBG
D. TBPA
REF: 33-p. 109

882. In the hyperthyroid patient, the number of available TBG binding sites is
A. decreased
B. increased
C. normal
REF: 1-p. 393

883. Estrogens increase the number of available binding sites on the plasma carrier proteins. Therefore, a T3 resin uptake will be falsely
A. elevated
B. depressed
C. normal
REF: 1-p. 393

884. Which of the following medications or conditions will result in falsely depressed T3 uptake values?
A. Heparin
B. Pregnancy
C. Oral contraceptives
D. All of the above
E. B and C only
REF: 39-p. 12

885. An elevated T3 uptake level can result from
A. true hyperthyroidism
B. factitious hypothyroidism
C. an increase in binding plasma proteins
D. a decrease in binding plasma proteins
E. A and C
F. A and D
REF: 33-p. 110

886. The purpose of the ethanol extraction step in the Murphy-Patee T4 analysis is to
A. bind free T4 to TBG
B. free bound T4 from TBG
C. bind free T3 to TBG
D. free bound T3 from TBG
E. A and C only
F. B and D only
REF: 32-p. 251

887. Drugs which falsely elevate serum T4 result in an otherwise euthyroid patient include all of the following EXCEPT
A. heparin
B. estrogens
C. Levodopa
D. oral contraceptives
REF: 1-p. 396

888. Conditions (such as pregnancy) or drugs (such as estrogens) which increase the amount of circulating TBG, will affect a serum T4 level by
A. decreasing it
B. elevating it
C. normalizing it
REF: 37-p. 100

889. Perturbations of the thyroid hormone-binding protein interaction may alter the results of which of the following in vitro thyroid tests?
A. Triiodothyronine uptake
B. Total serum thyroxine
C. TSH RIA
D. T3 RIA
E. All of the above
F. A and B only
REF: 37-p. 100

890. In cases of variations in TBG capacity, the true status of the thyroid gland can be accurately estimated using the
A. T3 uptake test
B. total T4 test
C. FT_4I determination
D. PBI determination
REF: 33-p. 112

891. The iodine conversion ratio test measures the amount of radioiodine bound to
A. erythrocytes
B. plasma proteins
C. thyroglobulin
D. all of the above
REF: 39-p. 13

892. The Free Thyroxine Index (FTI) was developed to adequately reflect thyroid status more so than the T3 uptake or the T4 test could do alone. This value is calculated using which of the following formulas?
A. $\frac{\text{T3 uptake}}{\text{T4}}$
B. $\frac{\text{T4}}{\text{T3 uptake}}$
C. T3 uptake x T4
D. T3 uptake x TBG
REF: 1-p. 394

893. Iodinated contrast materials adversely affect the results of all of the following EXCEPT
A. protein bound iodine analysis (PBI)
B. triiodothyronine uptake test (T3U)
C. butanol extractable iodine (BEI)
D. T4 by column
REF: 33-p. 106

894. The presence of circulating LATS (long-acting thyroid stimulator) may be indicative of which of the following thyroid conditions?

A. Graves' disease
B. Toxic nodular goiter
C. Thyroiditis
D. All of the above
E. A and C only
REF: 32-p. 252

13. CENTRAL NERVOUS SYSTEM

DIRECTIONS: Each of the questions or incomplete statements below is followed by a list of suggested answers or completions. Select the **one** that is **BEST** in each case.

---

895. The central nervous system (CNS) is made up of the
  A. brain
  B. spinal cord
  C. cranial nerves
  D. A and B
  E. A and C
  F. all of the above
  REF: 22-p. 7

896. The largest structure in the brain is the
  A. cerebellum
  B. cerebrum
  C. pons
  D. medulla
  E. corpus callosum
  REF: 1-p. 408

897. The two cerebral hemispheres are each divided into ____________ lobes.
A. 2
B. 3
C. 4
D. 5
E. 6
REF: 1-p. 408

898. The dural sinuses within the brain are responsible for
A. draining venous blood from the brain
B. supplying oxygenated blood to the brain
C. bathing the brain in cerebrospinal fluid
D. providing protection for cerebral arteries
E. acting as an arterial blood pool reservoir
REF: 32-p. 215

899. The point at which the superior sagittal and transverse sinuses of the brain join is the
A. pia mater
B. pons
C. cerebrospinal axis
D. fornix
E. confluence
REF: 51-p. 6

900. The lobe occupying the middle third of the external cerebral hemisphere enclosed by the Sylvian and Rolando fissure is the
A. parietal
B. frontal
C. quadrate
D. occipital
E. temporal
REF: 16-p. 645

901. Cerebrospinal fluid (CSF) is produced within the
A. cerebellum
B. basal ganglia
C. pons
D. spinal cord
E. choroid plexus
REF: 32-p. 215

902. The ventricle system of the brain is composed of ____________ cavities.
A. 2
B. 3
C. 4
D. 5
E. 6
REF: 1-p. 412

903. The total cerebrospinal fluid (CSF) in an adult is
A. 40 50 cc
B. 120-150 cc
C. 250-280 cc
D. 400-430 cc
E. 550-580 cc
REF: 47-p. 71

904. Cerebral spinal fluid leaves the ventricular system via the
A. inferior horns of the lateral ventricles
B. aqueduct of Sylvius
C. fourth ventricle
D. posterior horns of the lateral ventricles
E. interventricular formen
REF: 32-p. 226

905. At the upper portion of the thyroid cartilage, the common carotid arteries bifurcate into the
A. middle and posterior arteries
B. internal and external carotid arteries
C. anterior cerebral and middle arteries
D. external carotid and middle artery
E. basal and posterior arteries
REF: 32-p. 215

906. The internal carotid artery supplies blood to the cerebral hemispheres via the
A. anterior cerebral artery
B. middle cerebral artery
C. posterior cerebral artery
D. A and B
E. B and C
F. all of the above
REF: 32-p. 215

907. The term "blood-brain barrier" refers to the fact that
A. blood is filtered as it leaves the brain
B. the brain is impervious to insterstitial fluids
C. red blood cells do not have direct access to the brain
D. the brain vasculature is impermeable to proteins and most drugs
E. only blood may enter the brain
REF: 1-p. 415

908. The passage of substances across the blood-brain barrier is accomplished primarily by
A. passive diffusion
B. phagocytosis
C. pinocytosis
D. active transport
E. capillary transport
REF: 50-p. 55

909. In pediatric patients, 75% of all primary brain lesions occur in the
A. lateral ventricles
B. sagittal sinus
C. posterior fossa
D. frontal lobe
E. middle cerebral arteries
REF: 47-p. 57

910. The most common general class of tumors detectable by brain scintigraphy is the
A. metastatic
B. glioma
C. meningioma
D. pituitary
E. neurinoma
REF: 32-p. 221

911. All of the following are advantages of the use of radionuclide brain scintigraphy over the use of computed tomography as a screening method for detecting brain lesions EXCEPT that brain scintigraphy

A. can be accomplished at the patient's bedside
B. is less expensive
C. provides better anatomic detail
D. is less invasive
E. is better suited for providing physiologic information
REF: 38-p. 104

912. Brain scintigraphy using a ^{99m} technetium labeled radiopharmaceutical is indicated for all the following EXCEPT

A. subdural hematoma
B. meningioma
C. cerebral spinal fluid leak
D. cerebrovascular accident
E. arteriovenous malformation
REF: 17-p. 2

913. Patients with suspected ____________, should not undergo brain scintigraphy until at least 7 days after insult.

A. neoplasm
B. subdural hematoma
C. cerebral infarction
D. metastatic carcinoma
E. encephalitis
REF: 36-p. 401

914. When used for brain scintigraphy, $^{99m}TcO^{-}{}_4$ may be administered

A. intravenously
B. intramuscularly
C. orally
D. A and B
E. A and C
F. all of the above
REF: 47-p. 52

915. A ____________ scan accomplished within 48 hours before brain scintigraphy using $^{99m}TcO^-_4$ may cause a false-negative brain scan.

A. bone
B. liver
C. lung
D. renal
E. thyroid
REF: 47-p. 52

916. In normal physiologic conditions $^{99m}TcO^-_4$ accumulates in all the following sites EXCEPT the

A. gastric mucosa
B. thyroid gland
C. brain
D. salivary glands
E. urine
REF: 17-p. 3

917. The typical dose of $^{99m}TcO^-_4$ used for routine brain scintigraphy is

A. 0.5–1.0 mCi
B. 3.0–5.0 mCi
C. 5.0–10.0 mCi
D. 15.0–20.0 mCi
E. 25.0–30.0 mCi
REF: 36-p. 385

918. One of the main disadvantages of the use of $^{99m}TcO^-_4$ as a radiopharmaceutical for brain scintigraphy is that it

A. is relatively costly and difficult to obtain
B. localizes in the choroid plexus
C. does not effectively localize in most brain pathologies
D. readily localizes in the venous sinuses
E. precludes the use of relatively high doses due to its ionic extracellular distribution pattern
REF: 1-p. 416

919. The administration of 250 mg of potassium perchlorate prior to ^{99m}Tc pertechnetate injection in brain scintigraphy restricts radiopharmaceutical uptake in the
A. thyroid gland
B. choroid plexus
C. salivary glands
D. A and B
E. B and C
F. all of the above
REF: 50-p. 57

920. The patient preparation(s) for ^{99m}Tc DTPA brain scintigraphy is (are)
A. 200 mg potassium perchlorate 1 hour before the radiopharmaceutical is injected
B. thorough explanation of the procedure to the patient
C. at least 6 hours prior NPO orders
D. A and B
E. B and C
F. all of the above
REF: 36-p. 395

921. The usual time per image frame for adult cerebral radionuclide angiography is
A. 2 seconds
B. 4 seconds
C. 6 seconds
D. 8 seconds
E. 10 seconds
REF: 36-p. 385

922. The arterial phase on normal cerebral radionuclide angiography usually appears ____________ seconds after radiopharmaceutical administration and lasts approximately ____________ seconds.
A. 9; 6
B. 9; 12
C. 9; 18
D. 15; 6
E. 15; 12
REF: 49-p. 7

923. The signal for the end of capillary flush phase on an anterior cerebral radionuclide angiogram occurs when
A. the common carotid arteries are visualized
B. the venous sinus system is visualized
C. the cerebral arteries are visualized
D. oral activity appears
E. orbital activity appears
REF: 1-p. 418

924. The usual head position for adults in routine cerebral radionuclide angiography is the
A. anterior
B. posterior
C. vertex
D. Towne's
E. reverse Towne's
REF: 36-p. 386

925. In cerebral radionuclide angiography, the gamma camera should be started at about ___________ seconds after peripheral intravenous radiopharmaceutical administration.
A. 1-2
B. 6-8
C. 12-14
D. 20-24
E. 30-34
REF: 32-p. 219

926. The best way to increase the relatively poor statistics of a cerebral radionuclide angiogram using a ^{99m} technetium labeled radiopharmaceutical is to
A. hydrate the patient before injection
B. use multiple intravenous injections
C. employ a high sensitivity low energy collimator
D. block the choroid plexus with potassium perchlorate
E. open the camera's pulse height analyzer to 50%
REF: 36-p. 385

927. Activity on an abnormal cerebral radionuclide angiogram may appear as being
A. absent
B. decreased
C. increased
D. A and B
E. B and C
F. all of the above
REF: 36-p. 387

928. All of the following will produce a localized reduced perfusion appearance on a cerebral radionuclide angiogram EXCEPT
A. traumatic edema
B. subdural hematoma
C. cerebral embolism
D. meningioma
E. atherosclerosis
REF: 47-p. 58

929. A positive finding of cerebral death on an anterior cerebral radionuclide angiogram is made when the tracer bolus
A. immediately appears in the tranverse sinus
B. stops at the base of the skull without evidence of intracranial entry
C. is visualized in the middle cerebral artery but nonvisualized in the posterior cerebral artery
D. "hangs up" in the arterial phase of the cerebral arteries
E. bypasses the arterial phase and immediately enters the venous phase
REF: 47-p. 65

930. If peripheral veins are inaccessible for brain scintigraphy using $^{99}TcO^{-}{}_4$ in a pediatric patient, the radiopharmaceutical may be administered
A. topically
B. through a scalp vein
C. intraperitoneally
D. subcutaneously
E. via lumbar puncture
REF: 5-2(4):329, 1972

931. The usual number of counts for static brain scintigraphy is

A. 50,000-100,000
B. 100,000-200,000
C. 300,000-500,000
D. 500,000-750,000
E. 750,000-1,000,000
REF: 36-p. 394

932. Besides the anterior, posterior, and both laterals, the view(s) most often accomplished in routine static brain scintigraphy is (are) the

A. left and right anterior obliques
B. left and right posterior obliques
C. Towne's position
D. reverse Towne's position
E. vertex
REF: 49-p. 5

933. As a general rule, a lesion should be seen on _________ view(s) before the brain scan is considered positive.

A. one
B. at least two
C. at least three
D. the anterior
E. all
REF: 42-p. 5

934. Immediate ^{99}Tc pertechnetate static brain images show vascular details

A. exclusively
B. very prominently but less so in delayed images
C. very poorly but increasing over time
D. not at all but somewhat over time
E. not at all at any point in time
REF: 50-p. 57

935. On a normal anterior static brain image, the midline band of activity extending from the apex to the high activity region of the base of the skull represents
A. scalp activity
B. a midline skull fracture
C. superior sagittal sinus
D. occipital sinus
E. temporalis muscle
REF: 51-p. 4

936. Metastatic brain tumors usually appear on brain scintigrams
A. singularly
B. in multiple sites
C. as "cold" lesions
D. as "hot" lesions with "cold" centers
E. only in the rarest occasions
REF: 1-p. 419

937. The "doughnut" sign is most likely seen on static brain scans with patients having a (an)
A. burr hole
B. glioblastoma
C. aneurysm
D. arteriovenous shunt
E. meningioma
REF: 50-p. 64

938. The finding of a prominent right transverse sinus on a posterior static brain image most likely is a
A. normal variant
B. metastatic lesion
C. contamination spill on the patient
D. glioma
E. meningioma
REF: 50-p. 60

939. Brain abscesses are better detected with brain scintigraphy if
A. a radionuclide angiogram precedes static imaging
B. a vertex view is accomplished during static imaging
C. the usual dose of the radiopharmaceutical is doubled
D. high sensitivity gamma camera collimation is used
E. static imaging is delayed for 3 hours or longer
REF: 32-p. 223

940. Positron emission tomography (PET) imaging of the brain requires the use of
A. high sensitivity collimation
B. dual radiopharmaceutical administration
C. diametrically opposed detectors
D. high count rate capability probe systems
E. a computerized axial tomography (CAT) scanner
REF: 12-p. 323

941. The conclusive diagnostic exams for adult normal pressure hydrocephalus is
A. computerized tomography
B. sonography
C. radionuclide cisternography
D. pneumoencephalography
E. skull radiographic series
REF: 46-p. 127

942. Radionuclide cisternography is used for determination of all of the following EXCEPT
A. cerebral spinal fluid leaks
B. communicating hydrocephalus
C. spinal blocks
D. malignancy of the choroid plexus
E. ventricular shunt patency
REF: 52-p. 38

943. The radiopharmaceutical(s) used in radionuclide cisternography for the diagnosis of normal pressure hydrocephalus is (are)

A. ^{99m}Tc DTPA
B. ^{111}In DTPA
C. ^{169}Yb DTPA
D. A and B
E. B and C
F. all of the above
REF: 38-p. 113

944. The radiopharmaceutical is always administered ____________ in a radionuclide cisternogram.

A. intrathecally
B. intravenously
C. intraparietally
D. intraperitoneally
E. intrarterially
REF: 32-p. 227

945. The usual adult dose of either ^{169}Yb DTPA or ^{111}In DTPA for cisternography is

A. 100 mCi
B. 500 μCi
C. 2-3 mCi
D. 4-6 mCi
E. 8-10 mCi
REF: 49-p. 9

946. Besides using a "point" source for film indication of anatomical landmarks in radionuclide cisternography, a ____________ source is also commonly used.

A. calibration
B. plastic tubing
C. rod
D. commercial sheet
E. check
REF: 49-p. 13

947. In routine radionuclide cisternography to evaluate CSF flow, images are taken immediately, 4-6 hours, and
A. 12 and 18 hours
B. 12 and 24 hours
C. 24 and 48 hours
D. 24 and 72 hours
E. 48 and 72 hours
REF: 38-p. 114

948. The lumbar injection site is immediately scanned after radiopharmaceutical injection in radionuclide cisternography to
A. determine if the instillation was adequate
B. provide a baseline for the rate of CSF flow
C. determine the count statistics to be used in later imaging
D. check for any previous radiopharmaceutical administration
E. check for the integrity of the radiopharmaceutical
REF: 32-p. 227

949. In a normal 24-hour radionuclide cisternogram, there is ____________ activity within the ventricles.
A. no
B. little
C. diffuse
D. focal
E. intense
REF: 38-p. 115

950. The most common finding(s) of an abnormal 24-hour cisternogram besides a focus of decreased or increased radioactivity is (are)
A. nonvisualization of the cerebral convexities
B. visualization of the basal cisterns
C. visualization of the ventricles
D. A and B
E. B and C
F. A and C
REF: 17-p. 46

951. A technical aid for the detection of CSF rhinorrhea by radionuclide cisternography is to

A. hydrate the patient before injection
B. have the patient ambulate as long as possible after radiopharmaceutical administration
C. use a sensitive counting probe to localize the site of leakage
D. inject the radiopharmaceutical directly into the leakage site
E. pack the patient's nose with cotton pledgets before dose administration

REF: 53-p. 46

14. LIVER-SPLEEN

DIRECTIONS: Each of the questions or incomplete statements below is followed by a list of suggested answers or completions. Select the **one** that is **BEST** in each case.

---

952. The normal liver has ____________ blood supply.

A. only a venous
B. a dual portal vein & hepatic artery
C. a minimal
D. a variable
E. a positional dependent
REF: 50-p. 153

953. Sugar is stored in the liver in the form of

A. glucose
B. fructose
C. maltose
D. glycogen
E. glycine
REF: 22-p. 26

954. The organ(s) most susceptible to injury from blunt trauma is (are) the
A. liver
B. spleen
C. kidneys
D. heart
E. lungs
REF: 38-p. 257

955. A normal variation of the extension of the right lobe of the liver to the level of the umbilicus or below as seen on liver scintigraphy is most likely due to
A. removal of the spleen
B. Riedel's lobe
C. kidney indentation
D. a prominent gallbladder fossa
E. Liebermeister's groove
REF: 15-p. 8

956. The liver usually becomes enlarged if the patient is known to have
A. a hepatic hematoma
B. hepatic metastases
C. advanced hepatitis
D. a hepatoma
E. a hepatic cyst
REF: 17-p. 66

957. Approximately ____________% of all liver cells are Kupffer cells.
A. 15
B. 30
C. 45
D. 60
E. 75
REF: 32-p. 330

958. The polygonal cells or hepatocytes of the liver function in all of the following EXCEPT
A. carbohydrate metabolism
B. foreign matter phagocytosis Kupffer
C. vitamin storage
D. fatty acid kinetics
E. protein synthesis
REF: 32-p. 330

959. The spleen is normally a hematopoietic organ during
A. fetal life
B. neonate life
C. early childhood
D. adolescence
E. adult life
REF: 15-p. 245

960. The normal adult spleen as determined by the posterior image on ^{99m}Tc sulfur colloid scintigraphy is about ____________ cm ± 1.5 cm.
A. 5
B. 10
C. 15
D. 20
E. 25
REF: 4-12:123, 1971

961. Bile is
A. produced in the gallbladder (liver)
B. stored in the liver
C. extracted from the blood stream
D. produced in the common duct
E. stored in the gallbladder
REF: 22-p. 27

962. Nuclear medicine techniques for liver scintigraphy include the use of (a) radiopharmaceutical(s) that is (are)
- **A.** cleared by the polygonal cells and secreted into the biliary system
- **B.** mechanically trapped within the liver's capillary system
- **C.** phagocytized by the reticuloendothelical (RE) cells
- **D.** A and B
- **E.** A and C
- **F.** B and C

REF: 14-p. 1

Kuppfer

963. The radiopharmaceutical of choice for imaging the RE system of the liver with a gamma camera is
- **A.** ^{113m}In hydroxide
- **B.** ^{99m}Tc sulfur colloid
- **C.** ^{198}Au colloid
- **D.** ^{99m}Tc MAA
- **E.** ^{99m}Tc red blood cells

REF: 14-p. 2

964. The average recommended adult dose of ^{99m}Tc sulfur colloid for routine liver spleen scintigraphy is
- **A.** 1 mCi
- **B.** 3 mCi
- **C.** 5 mCi
- **D.** 10 mCi
- **E.** 20 mCi

REF: 14-p. 3

965. The maximum clearance of colloid particles in a single pass through normal adult liver is approximately
- **A.** 35%
- **B.** 50%
- **C.** 65%
- **D.** 80%
- **E.** 95%

REF: 50-p. 155

966. Within 15 minutes after injection, ____________% of ^{99m}Tc sulfur colloid is localized within the liver in a normal patient.
A. 10–20
B. 30–40
C. 40–50
D. 60–70
E. 80–90
REF: 33-p. 132

967. There should be a delay of at least ____________ following administration of ^{99m}Tc sulfur colloid before liver imaging begins.
A. 2 minutes
B. 15 minutes
C. 45 minutes
D. 1 hour
E. 2 hours
REF: 14-p. 3

968. The range of diameter size of ^{99m}Tc sulfur colloid particles is
A. 0.1 millimicron to 1.0 millimicron
B. 0.1 millimicron to 1.0 micron
C. 0.1 millimicron to 1.0 millimeter
D. 0.1 micron to 1.0 millimeter
E. 0.1 micron to 10.0 millimeters
REF: 1-p. 558

969. The presence of overly large ^{99m}Tc sulfur colloid particles (> 1.0 micron) may be detected on a scan when there is
A. exclusive splenic uptake
B. excessive lung activity
C. visualization of the thyroid
D. lack of bone marrow activity
E. rapid turnover of liver activity
REF: 55-p. 143

970. If the mean particle size of ^{99m}Tc sulfur colloid particles is reduced, the biodistribution would be altered by
A. less localization in the spleen and more in bone marrow
B. less localization in the spleen and more in the liver
C. more localization in the spleen and less in bone marrow
D. more localization in the spleen and less in the liver
E. more in both the spleen and the liver
REF: 1-p. 559

971. All of the following are indications for ^{99m}Tc sulfur colloid liver scintigraphy EXCEPT
A. evaluation of liver size and shape
B. localization of hepatic lesions for biopsy
C. quantification of hepatic artery blood flow rate
D. evaluation of diffuse hepatic disease such as hepatitis or cirrhosis
E. detection of lesions such as hematoma, tumor, or abscess
REF: 17-p. 61

972. Abnormal liver lesions appear on ^{99m}Tc sulfur colloid scintigraphy often as
A. focal "cold" areas
B. focal and diffuse "cold" areas
C. focal "hot" areas
D. focal and diffuse "hot" areas
E. focal "hot" or "cold" areas
REF: 1-p. 453

973. The appearance of the normal liver on dynamic scintigraphy of the liver occurs
A. several seconds before lung visualization
B. at the same time as lung visualization
C. several seconds after lung visualization
D. at the same time as kidney and spleen visualization
E. several seconds after kidney and spleen visualization
REF: 15-p. 79

974. Dynamic imaging of the liver using ^{99m}Tc sulfur colloid should be carried out for at least
A. 10-15 seconds
B. 30-35 seconds
C. 50-60 seconds
D. 2-3 minutes
E. 4-5 minutes
REF: 49-p. 45

975. A lineal lead marker of known size placed over the left costal margin on the anterior image of a liver spleen scintigram aids in determining liver
A. size
B. position
C. function
D. A and B
E. B and C
F. all of the above
REF: 14-p. 4

976. If a GI tract barium study is performed before ^{99m}Tc sulfur colloid scintigraphy, the patient must
A. have an administration of double the usual radiopharmaceutical dose
B. be well hydrated
C. have the study postponed for 1 week
D. be imaged with the inspiration or expiration method
E. have a cleansing enema before being injected with the radiopharmaceutical
REF: 49-p. 49

977. Normal areas of decreased activity occurring on an anterior ^{99m}Tc sulfur colloid liver image include
A. right kidney indentation
B. porta hepatis
C. gallbladder fossa
D. A and B
E. B and C
F. all of the above
REF: 17-p. 64

978. On an anterior image of a ^{99m}Tc sulfur colloid liver scan, the right and left lobes of the liver are usually
- **A.** overlapped and therefore not readily separated
- **B.** clearly separated by the porta hepatis
- **C.** separated by overlying sternum
- **D.** distinguished by increased border activity
- **E.** distinguished by increased activity appearing in the left lobe

REF: 17-p. 64

979. If at all possible, every patient having a ^{99m}Tc sulfur colloid liver scan should have the anterior image obtained both in the supine and the ____________ position.
- **A.** standing
- **B.** prone
- **C.** sitting
- **D.** right side decubitis
- **E.** left side decubitis

REF: 4-18(11):1128, 1977

980. The best way to avoid a "cold" shadow artifact produced by pendulous breasts on a ^{99m}Tc sulfur colloid anterior liver image is to
- **A.** substitute both anterior obliques in lieu of the anterior image
- **B.** have patient stand during the anterior view
- **C.** position the patient in the right lateral decubitus position while obtaining the anterior image
- **D.** use a high information density setting in the region of the breast shadow
- **E.** instruct the patient to elevate her breasts during the view

REF: 14-p. 11

981. Advanced cirrhosis of the liver on ^{99m}Tc sulfur colloid exams appear as having a (an)
- **A.** patchy, diffuse appearance
- **B.** increased size of liver
- **C.** increased liver uptake of the radiopharmaceutical
- **D.** A and B
- **E.** B and C
- **F.** all of the above

REF: 17-p. 66

982. With severe hepatic disease, the radiation dose of ^{99m}Tc sulfur colloid to the ____________ is tripled.
A. whole body
B. testes/ovaries
C. bone marrow
D. liver
E. heart
REF: 33–p. 134

983. Radiation treatment (3000–3500 rads) to the liver characteristically produces a lesion on ^{99m}Tc sulfur colloid scintigraphy which appear as
A. a reversible area of significantly decreased activity
B. an irreversible area of significantly decreased activity
C. a reversible area of significantly increased activity
D. an irreversible area of significantly increased activity
E. an irreversible area of slightly increased activity
REF: 14–p. 25

984. Trauma-induced liver lacerations appear on ^{99m}Tc sulfur colloid scintigraphy as
A. patchy areas of decreased activity
B. a band of decreased activity
C. multifocal areas of decreased activity
D. a focal area of increased activity
E. either a focal area of increased or decreased activity depending upon the severity
REF: 17–p. 66

985. A hepatoma routinely concentrates
A. ^{198}Au colloid
B. ^{99m}Tc sulfur colloid
C. ^{67}Ga
D. ^{51}Cr red blood cells
E. ^{99m}Tc antimony colloid
REF: 15–p. 50

986. The rarely seen "hot spot" produced on ^{99m}Tc sulfur colloid liver scintigrams is most likely due to
A. radiation portal
B. extrahepatic mass
C. superior vena cava obstruction
D. "clumping" of the colloidal particles
E. polycystic liver disease
REF: 14–p. 26

987. ^{99m}Tc labeled bone-seeking radiopharmaceuticals will accumulate in abnormal liver tissue when
A. calcium-containing lesions are present
B. the radiolabel breaks down
C. liver perfusion is increased over normal levels
D. the cystic duct is obstructed
E. doses exceed 30 mCi
REF: 54–2:265, 1977

988. On a normal ^{99m}Tc sulfur colloid left lateral image the spleen lies ____________ (to) the liver.
A. superior
B. inferior
C. anterior
D. posterior
E. beneath
REF: 36–p. 496

989. Higher accumulation of ^{99m}Tc sulfur colloid in the spleen and to a lesser extent in bone marrow occurs in all of the following pathologies EXCEPT
A. metastatic carcinoma
B. Hodgkin's disease
C. congestive heart failure
D. polycythemia
E. cirrhosis
REF: 1–p. 455

990. ^{99m}Tc sulfur colloid scintigraphy of the spleen may evaluate or detect all of the following EXCEPT

A. splenic size
B. splenic shape
C. polygonal cell function
D. phagocytic functions
E. space-occupying lesions
REF: 36-p. 520

991. All of the following are known to cause splenomegaly EXCEPT

A. infiltrative disease
B. infectious disease (e.g., malaria)
C. damaged splenic blood supply
D. lymphoma
E. liver cirrhosis
REF: 15-p. 232

992. The spleen's size is best estimated on ^{99m}Tc sulfur colloid scintigraphy on the __________ view.

A. anterior
B. left anterior oblique
C. left lateral
D. left posterior oblique
E. posterior
REF: 36-p. 521

993. Besides the posterior and left lateral images, other views that should be accomplished in ^{99m}Tc sulfur colloid scintigraphy for evaluation of spleen trauma include

A. right lateral
B. right posterior oblique
C. left posterior oblique
D. A and B
E. B and C
F. all of the above
REF: 38-p. 258

994. The anatomic presence of a spleen without the ability to concentrate radioactive particles is termed
A. splenic anoxia
B. splenic shunting
C. functional asplenia
D. accessory splenic function
E. splenulus
REF: 15–p. 233

995. The spleen of a patient with severe chronic sickle cell disease on ^{99m}Tc sulfur colloid gamma camera images would probably be
A. enlarged but with homogenous activity
B. enlarged with multiple diffuse cold areas
C. displaced but with homogenous activity
D. displaced with multiple diffuse cold areas
E. nonvisualized
REF: 36–p. 523

996. Focal cold splenic defects appearing on ^{99m}Tc sulfur colloid liver–spleen scintigrams are rarely due to
A. infarction
B. cysts
C. metastatic cancer
D. contusion
E. hemorrhage
REF: 33–p. 140

997. Which one of the following radiopharmaceuticals will localize only in the spleen?
A. ^{99m}Tc sulfur colloid
B. ^{198}Au colloid
C. ^{99m}Tc denatured red blood cells
D. ^{113m}In colloid
E. ^{99m}Tc HIDA
REF: 52–p. 117

998. A nonimaging splenic sequestration study using ^{51}Cr red blood cells assesses the spleen's rate of
A. phagocytosis
B. erythrocyte destruction
C. hematopoiesis
D. blood elements accumulation
E. hormone production
REF: 15-p. 241

999. The nonimaging ^{51}Cr red blood cell spleen sequestration procedure involves external probe counting of the spleen and
A. liver
B. left kidney
C. precordium
D. A and B
E. A and C
F. all of the above
REF: 36-p. 294

1000. The normal ratio of spleen to liver activity derived from a ^{51}Cr red blood cell probe study is about
A. 0.5:1
B. 1:1
C. 2:1
D. 3:1
E. 4:1
REF: 36-p. 295

15. URINARY TRACT

DIRECTIONS: Each of the questions or incomplete statements below is followed by a list of suggested answers or completions. Select the **one** that is **BEST** in each case.

1001. One of the main functions of the kidney is to
- **A.** produce enzymes
- **B.** produce protein
- **C.** regulate body water
- **D.** maintain defense mechanism
- **E.** phagocytize cellular fragments

REF: 22-p. 129

1002. Kidney function is strongly influenced by
- **A.** antidiuretic hormone (ADH)
- **B.** erythropoietin
- **C.** thyroxine
- **D.** vasopressin
- **E.** pitressin

REF: 22-p. 132

1003. Renal blood flow in a normal resting man is approximately
A. 300 ml/min
B. 600 ml/min
C. 1200 ml/min
D. 2400 ml/min
E. 4800 ml/min
REF: 22-p. 130

1004. The functional unit of the kidney is the
A. nephron
B. glomerulus
C. Bowman's capsule
D. Henle's loop
E. proximal tubule
REF: 40-p. 129

1005. The cortex of the kidney contains the
A. calyces
B. ureter
C. glomerular capsules
D. renal pyramids
E. renal pelvis
REF: 16-p. 987

1006. The right kidney as compared to the left kidney in a normal patient is usually
A. slightly smaller
B. slightly larger
C. positioned somewhat lower
D. positioned somewhat higher
E. the same size and position
REF: 16-p. 985

1007. The three kidney processes involved in urine formation are glomerular filtration,
A. tubular contraction
B. tubular reabsorption
C. tubular excretion
D. A and B
E. A and C
F. B and C
REF: 32-p. 346

1008. The classic formula to calculate plasma clearance (C), with U being the concentration of a substance in the urine, P being the same substance in plasma, and V being the rate of urine flow is

A. $C = \frac{UV}{P}$
B. $C = \frac{PV}{U}$
C. $C = \frac{PU}{V}$
D. $C = \frac{V}{PU}$
E. $C = \frac{P}{UV}$
REF: 32-p. 345

1009. The normal adult glomerular filtration rate is

A. 25 ml/min
B. 50 ml/min
C. 100 ml/min
D. 125 ml/min
E. 150 ml/min
REF: 47-p. 249

1010. All of the following are valid reasons for renal scintigraphy EXCEPT

A. detection of renovascular hypertension
B. evaluation of renal artery morphology
C. evaluation of obstructive uropathies
D. delineation of renal masses
E. estimation of renal function
REF: 38-pp. 176-180

1011. The most efficacious diagnostic modality to evaluate a known renal mass is

A. intravenous pyelography
B. CAT scan
C. x-ray arteriography
D. grey-scale ultrasound
E. nuclear scintigraphy
REF: 38-p. 181

1012. ^{99cm}Technetium as pertechnetate used in renal scintigraphy should only be used to evaluate
A. tubular secretion
B. polycystic kidney disease
C. urinomas
D. renal perfusion
E. renal pelvic obstruction
REF: 47-p. 249

1013. All of the following radiopharmaceuticals will visualize the excretory system EXCEPT
A. ^{99cm}Tc DMSA
B. ^{99cm}Tc DTPA
C. ^{99cm}Tc GHA
D. ^{131}I Hippuran
E. ^{197}Hg chlormerodrin
REF: 36-p. 422

1014. Which of the following radiopharmaceuticals used in renal scintigraphy localize by a combination of glomerular filtration, tubular secretion, and tubular binding?
A. ^{131}I Hippuran
B. ^{197}Hg chlormerodrin
C. ^{99cm}Tc DTPA
D. ^{99cm}Tc GHA
E. ^{99cm}Tc DMSA
REF: 17-p. 138

1015. The localization mechanisms of all radiopharmaceuticals used for morphologic imaging of the kidneys are classified as those that
A. intensely localize in the presence of disease but otherwise are faint in the normal kidney
B. have a functional aspect but whose transit time is long enough to adequately image the kidneys
C. localize within the cortex
D. A and B
E. B and C
F. all of the above
REF: 38-p. 176

1016. Dynamic ^{131}I Hippuran scintigraphy is best used to evaluate
- **A.** renal tubular cell extraction and secretory function
- **B.** renal position and anatomy
- **C.** the extent of glomerulonephritis and pyelonephritis
- **D.** renal vascular disease
- **E.** obstructive uropathies

REF: 36-p. 422

1017. Renal artery disease evaluated by ^{131}I Hippuran scintigraphy appears in the affected kidney as
- **A.** a well-defined "cold" focal area that intensifies over time
- **B.** multiple focal "cold" areas that do not accumulate activity over time
- **C.** a patchy appearance that eventually becomes focally "cold"
- **D.** increased activity which is quickly removed from the kidney
- **E.** initial decreased activity which increases over time

REF: 36-p. 421

1018. Administration of 10 drops of Lugol's solution prior to ^{131}I Hippuran scintigraphy is recommended to
- **A.** increase the in vivo stability of ^{131}I Hippuran
- **B.** facilitate renal tubular uptake and excretion
- **C.** localize the kidneys prior to ^{131}I Hippuran administration
- **D.** block the uptake of free ^{131}I within the thyroid
- **E.** aid in the anatomical definition of the kidneys

REF: 36-p. 422

1019. About ____________% of ^{131}I Hippuran localizes in the urine of a normal patient by tubular secretion.
- **A.** 15
- **B.** 30
- **C.** 55
- **D.** 80
- **E.** 95

REF: 47-p. 249

1020. Peak concentration of ^{131}I Hippuran within a normal kidney appears at ____________ minutes while the majority of activity is localized in the bladder at the end of ____________ minutes.

A. 1–2; 10
B. 1–2; 20
C. 1–2; 30
D. 4–6; 10
E. 4–6; 20
REF: 36–p. 423

1021. The critical organ in the ^{131}I Hippuran procedure is the

A. bladder
B. kidney
C. ureter
D. gonad
E. thyroid
REF: 47–p. 250

1022. Which of the following is (are) a part of renal evaluation in a radionuclide renogram?

A. Blood flow
B. Radionuclide extraction
C. Radionuclide excretion
D. A and B
E. B and C
F. All of the above
REF: 36–p. 419

1023. Besides a background correction, computer analysis of a ^{131}I Hippuran study also usually requires a correction for

A. renal size
B. renal location
C. renal motion
D. previously administered ^{99cm}Tc DTPA
E. extravasated dose
REF: 53–p. 183

1024. The initial rise in counts seen on a camera/computer-generated renogram within 30 seconds after administration of ^{131}I Hippuran constitutes the ___________ phase.

A. vascular
B. cortical
C. collecting
D. secretory
E. excretory
REF: 53-p. 184

1025. Prolonged bilateral transit time and reduced excretion noted on a computer-generated ^{131}I Hippuran may be due to a patient with poor cardiac output or who

A. is dehydrated
B. is overhydrated
C. is obese
D. has a full bladder
E. has been given a diuretic
REF: 53-p. 184

1026. The principal advantage(s) of a commercially produced ^{123}I Hippuran over ^{131}I Hippuran is (are) the ^{123}I preparation would

A. deliver a lower radiation dose to the patient
B. be better imaged with today's gamma camera
C. cost less in routine use
D. A and B
E. B and C
F. all of the above
REF: 58-p. 331

1027. The ^{131}I Hippuran study always follows the ^{99m}Tc DTPA when evaluating both glomerular function and tubular secretion because
A. the ^{99m}Tc DTPA enhances the tubular secretion of ^{131}I Hippuran
B. the 360 keV photopeak of ^{131}I will compromise the ^{99m}Tc DTPA by scattering into the 140 keV photopeak of ^{99m}Tc
C. any potential allergic ^{131}I reaction will first be determined by the less harmful ^{99m}Tc
D. the radiation dose delivered by ^{131}I will be significantly lessened if it can be bound and filtered with residual ^{99m}Tc DTPA
E. the ^{131}I Hippuran is the shorter of the two studies
REF: 47-p. 251

1028. The best radiopharmaceutical for evaluation of the renal cortex when there is no need for evaluation of the ureters and the bladder is
A. ^{99m}Tc DTPA
B. ^{99m}Tc DMSA
C. ^{99m}Tc GHA
D. ^{99m}Tc O^-_4
E. ^{131}I Hippuran
REF: 47-p. 251

1029. Shortly after introduction of ^{99m}Tc DMSA into the blood stream, it becomes
A. excreted by the kidneys
B. plasma bound
C. metabolized
D. filtered by the glomeruli
E. localized in the medulla
REF: 53-p. 181

1030. ^{99m}Tc DMSA renal uptake is proportional to both renal blood flow and
A. vascular disease
B. tubular function
C. glomerular function
D. renal configuration
E. glomerular filtration rate
REF: 36-p. 420

1031. The usual dose of ^{99m}Tc DMSA for static renal scintigraphy is
A. 500 μCi
B. 1-2 mCi
C. 5 mCi
D. 10 mCi
E. 20 mCi
REF: 36-p. 420

1032. A delay of ____________ is recommended after ^{99m}Tc DMSA patient administration before renal imaging is begun.
A. 15-20 minutes
B. 45-60 minutes
C. 1-2 hours
D. 2-3 hours
E. 4-6 hours
REF: 36-p. 420

1033. Static ^{99m}Tc DMSA scintigraphy accomplished on a gamma camera should have a minimum of __________ counts.
A. 50K
B. 100K
C. 300K
D. 700K
E. 1000K
REF: 32-p. 354

1034. Focally decreased areas on dynamic and static ^{99m}Tc DMSA renal images are typical findings in all of the following EXCEPT
A. polycystic disease
B. bacterial abscess
C. renal adenocarcinoma
D. infarcted cortex
E. metastatic lesion
REF: 53-p. 188

1035. ^{99m}Tc DMSA is not an ideal radiopharmaceutical to obtain dynamic images of the kidney because it

A. poorly delineates the kidneys
B. is significantly and efficiently accumulated in the liver in the first few transits
C. does not follow the usual tracer kinetics of perfusion agents
D. cannot be administered in dosages high enough for short duration images with adequate statistics
E. cannot be made in concentrations suitable for a bolus administration technique

REF: 58-p. 329

1036. To help improve the qualitative evaluation of renal cortex anatomy with either ^{99m}Tc GHA or ^{99m}Tc DMSA, the technologist should

A. improve the counting statistics by administering double the usual adult dose
B. obtain posterior oblique and lateral images
C. use a pinhole collimator to obtain magnified images
D. A and B
E. B and C
F. all of the above

REF: 58-p. 341

1037. The easiest way to achieve the same renal cortex concentration of ^{99m}Tc GHA as can be obtained by ^{99m}Tc DMSA is to

A. increase the administered dose of ^{99m}Tc GHA
B. slightly oxidize the ^{99m}Tc GHA prior to administration
C. hydrate the patient for 6 hours prior to scintigraphy
D. stress the patient on a treadmill just prior to scintigraphy
E. administer a mild diuretic to the patient within 15 minutes of radiopharmaceutical administration

REF: 58-p. 330

1038. The best radiopharmaceutical for quantification of the glomerular rate (GFR) is
A. ^{99m}Tc DMSA
B. ^{99m}Tc DTPA
C. ^{99m}Tc GHA
D. ^{99m}Tc FeA
E. $^{99m}TcO_4^-$
REF: 58-p. 329

1039. ^{99cm}Tc DTPA used in renal scintigraphy is best suited for evaluation of
A. renal parenchyma
B. renal plasma flow
C. renal vascular flow
D. renal insufficiency
E. renal size
REF: 53-p. 180

1040. The transport mechanism of ^{99m}Tc DTPA through the glomerular structure of kidney is termed
A. passive filtration
B. mechanical blocking
C. tubular secretion
D. active transport
E. semiactive secretion
REF: 47-p. 248

1041. The typical adult dose of ^{99m}Tc DTPA used for dynamic renal scintigraphy is
A. 0.5-1 mCi
B. 1-3 mCi
C. 5-10 mCi
D. 10-15 mCi
E. 20-25 mCi
REF: 32-p. 354

1042. Sequential renal imaging with ^{99m}Tc DTPA is best performed on a ____________ gamma camera equipped with a ____________ collimator.
A. standard field of view; parallel hole
B. standard field of view; pinhold
C. standard field of view; diverging
D. large field of view; parallel
E. large field of view; diverging
REF: 32-p. 340

1043. Optimal static ^{99m}Tc DTPA images of the renal cortex are obtained at ____________ after administration.
A. 30 seconds
B. 3–5 minutes
C. 20–30 minutes
D. 1–2 hours
E. 3–4 hours
REF: 53-p. 187

1044. A finding of acute pyelonephritis typically appears on ^{99m}Tc DTPA static scintigraphy as
A. normal sized kidneys with multifocal cold defects
B. normal sized kidneys with generalized decreased activity
C. enlarged kidneys with markedly increased activity
D. enlarged kidneys with generalized decreased activity
E. either normal or enlarged kidneys with markedly increased activity
REF: 53-p. 188

1045. A renal dynamic study using a bolus of ^{99m}Tc DTPA should be acquired on a gamma camera for ____________ seconds/frame and on a computer for ____________ seconds/frame for a total of about 30 seconds after activity is seen in the descending aorta.
A. 0.5 to 1; 0.5 to 1
B. 2 to 5; 0.5 to 1
C. 2 to 5; 2 to 5
D. 5 to 8; 2 to 5
E. 5 to 8; 5 to 8
REF: 32-p. 354

1046. The arrival of a compact bolus of ^{99m}Tc DTPA at the kidneys on normal dynamic scintigraphy should be noted by

A. first vascular blush on the right, then predominance of activity on the right
B. first vascular blush on the right, then predominance of activity on the left
C. first vascular blush on the left, then predominance of activity on the right
D. first vascular blush on the left, then predominance of activity on the left
E. simultaneous left and right vascular blush, then symmetric activity of equal intensity
REF: 17-p. 140

1047. A decreased renal perfusion asymmetry noted on a ^{99m}Tc DTPA dynamic study most likely suggests unilateral

A. AVM
B. acute obstructive uropathy
C. renal contusion
D. renal vein thrombosis
E. renal artery stenosis
REF: 53-p. 188

1048. The diuretic lasix, administered after findings of hydroureteronephrosis on ^{99m}Tc DTPA scintigrams, is used to distinguish benign dilated systems from those that have

A. lacerated ureters
B. ureter reflux
C. mechanical obstruction
D. poor excretion
E. slowed filtration
REF: 5-11:89, 1981

1049. Lasix can be administered to a pediatric patient after ^{99m}Tc DTPA images demonstrate hydronephrosis only after the patient
A. is ambulated for 30 minutes
B. voids prior to lasix administration
C. is NPO for at least 6 hours
D. eats a fatty meal
E. receives a second dose of ^{99m}Tc DTPA
REF: 4-20(6):622, 1979

1050. The usual patient positioning for dynamic and static scintigraphy of a transplanted kidney is
A. supine, anterior
B. supine, posterior
C. prone, anterior
D. prone, posterior
E. upright, posterior
REF: 47-p. 251

1051. The typical adult dose of ^{131}I Hippuran for scintigraphic evaluation of the transplanted kidney is
A. 50 mCi
B. 200 mCi
C. 750 mCi
D. 1 mCi
E. 2 mCi
REF: 4-20(10):1029, 1979

1052. Initial ^{99m}Tc DTPA and ^{131}I Hippuran scintigraphic evaluations of a transplanted kidney are typically first performed
A. within 24 hours following surgery
B. within 1 week after surgery
C. when urine production ceases
D. when ATN is suspected
E. when creatinine and urea blood levels become elevated
REF: 4-20(10):1029, 1979

1053. The radiopharmaceutical of choice to evaluate early renal graft rejection noted by its significant uptake within the kidney is
A. ^{67}Ga
B. ^{131}I fibrinogen
C. ^{99m}Tc DMSA
D. ^{99m}Tc MDP
E. ^{99m}Tc sulfur colloid
REF: 4-17:175, 1976

1054. Acute rejection of a transplanted kidney detected by nuclear scintigraphy appears as ____________ activity on the ^{99m}Tc DTPA dynamic images and ____________ activity on the ^{131}I Hippuran images.
A. normal; delayed
B. absent; normal
C. absent; delayed
D. delayed; diminished
E. diminished; normal
REF: 4-16:1115, 1975

1055. Vesicoureteral reflux in children may be detected by
A. a catheterized bladder radiographic technique
B. a catheterized bladder radionuclidic technique
C. a noncatheterized bladder radionuclidic technique
D. A and B
E. A and C
F. all of the above
REF: 58-p. 367

1056. All of the following are advantages of nuclear cystography over the comparable x-ray procedure EXCEPT the radionuclidic study
A. can be quantitated with the use of a minicomputer
B. is sensitive for even minimal reflux
C. delivers a considerably lower radiation
D. provides greater anatomic detail
E. uses nonallergenic agents
REF: 17-p. 158

1057. Typical pediatric doses of $^{99m}TcO_4^-$ radionuclide cystography are
A. 1–2 mCi
B. 3–5 mCi
C. 8–10 mCi
D. 10–12 mCi
E. 12–15 mCi
REF: 17–p. 158

1058. The proper patient positioning for the filling phase of direct nuclear cystography is the patient being
A. upright with the bladder on the top of the field of view
B. upright with the entire bladder centered in the field of view
C. upright with the upper half of the bladder in the bottom of field of view
D. supine with the bladder on the top of the field of view
E. supine with the entire bladder centered in the field of view
F. supine with the upper half of the bladder on the bottom of the field of view
REF: 32–p. 359

1059. After the bladder is filled to capacity during direct radionuclidic cystography, acquisition of 300,000 count images of the urinary tract begins in which of the following positions?
A. Anterior
B. Posterior
C. Anterior, left and right anterior obliques
D. Posterior, left and right posterior obliques
E. Anterior, posterior, left and right anterior and posterior obliques
REF: 32–p. 359

1060. The advantage of the indirect method of radionuclide cystography over the direct method is that the indirect method

A. can detect reflux during the filling phase of the bladder
B. does not require any cooperation of the patient
C. avoids bladder catheterization
D. accurately determines the bladder volume at which reflux occurs
E. has a lower background interference
REF: 58–p. 371

16. SKELETAL SYSTEM

DIRECTIONS: Each of the questions or incomplete statements below is followed by a list of suggested answers or completions. Select the **one** that is **BEST** in each case.

1061. Included in the axial portion of the skeleton are the thoracic cage, spine, and
A. skull
B. upper extremities
C. pelvis
D. femurs
E. humeri
REF: 47-p. 214

1062. The flat bones within the body are the
A. femurs, tibiae, and fibulae
B. carpals, sesamoids, and tarsals
C. scapulae, sternum, and ribs
D. spine, pelvis, and skull
E. metacarpals, phalanges, and metatarsals
REF: 32-p. 370

1063. The wrist, ankle, and sesamoid bones constitute the group of ____________ bones.
A. short
B. long
C. tubular
D. flat
E. irregular
REF: 32-p. 370

1064. The outer portion of all bones are covered by
A. articular cartilage
B. periosteum
C. compact bone
D. spongy bone
E. endosteum
REF: 32-p. 368

1065. Red bone marrow in normal healthy adults is found in the flat bones, vault of the skull, and
A. vertebrae
B. ends of long bones
C. mid shaft of long bones
D. A and B
E. A and C
F. B and C
REF: 1-p. 378

1066. Osteoblasts are most often located in
A. growing bones
B. decalcifying bones
C. cartilage and bone junction
D. healthy and stable bones
E. tumorous bone
REF: 22-p. 84

1067. Osteocytes, one of the three types of bone cells, are found in
A. growing bones
B. healthy stable bones
C. decalcifying bone
D. collagen
E. cartilage
REF: 22-p. 84

1068. Of the total body calcium, ____________% is found in the skeleton and ____________% is in the extracellular fluid and membranes.
A. 25; 75
B. 50; 50
C. 75; 25
D. 90; 10
E. 99; 1
REF: 1-p. 377

1069. Besides calcium, the crystalline lattice structure of bone is composed of
A. phosphate
B. carbon
C. hydroxyl ions
D. A and B
E. B and C
F. A and C
REF: 47-p. 214

1070. A bone loses ____________% of its calcium content before it is detectable on a ^{99m}Tc MDP bone scan.
A. A minimal
B. 20
C. 30
D. 50
E. 70
REF: 50-p. 117

1071. All of the following are ideal characteristics of a bone imaging agent except that the radiopharmaceutical should not have a (an)
A. immediate availability
B. slow soft tissue clearance
C. a high target-to-nontarget ratio
D. absence of adverse reaction
E. high extraction efficiency
REF: 50-p. 113

1072. ^{47}Ca has not found widespread use as a radionuclide for bone scintigraphy because it
A. does not behave similarly in the body to stable calcium
B. is a pure beta emitter and cannot penetrate tissue
C. cannot be "tagged" to any pharmaceutical
D. has an energy too high for nuclear medicine imaging instrumentation
E. is highly toxic in humans
REF: 1-p. 378

1073. The most commonly used radiopharmaceuticals for bone scintigraphy are composed of
A. analogs of calcium
B. calcium-rich compounds
C. analogs of phosphate
D. hydroxyl-rich compounds
E. analogs of strontium
REF: 47-p. 215

1074. The least satisfactory of all the ^{99m}Tc labeled phosphate analogs for routine bone scintigraphy is
A. MDP
B. MHDP
C. EHDP
D. PYP
E. HDP
REF: 47-p. 215

1075. The localization mechanism for the ^{99m}Tc phosphonate derivative bone agents is termed
A. chemisorption
B. active transport
C. mechanical blocking
D. pinocytosis
E. simple diffusion
REF: 54-6(10s):68, 1981

1076. The proposed factor which is the most important factor for ^{99m}Tc labeled phosphates to localize in pathologic sites of bone is thought to be
A. altered capillary permeability
B. altered metabolic activity
C. increased extraction efficiency
D. increased bone perfusion
E. decreased calcium content
REF: 50-p. 117

1077. The ^{99m}Tc labeled diphosphonate derivatives (e.g., EHDP, MDP, HMDP) used for skeletal scintigraphy contain stable ____________ bonds.
A. P—O
B. P—P
C. P—N—P
D. P—C—P
E. P—O—P
REF: 50-p. 110

1078. The organ receiving the greatest radiation dose using a ^{99m}Tc labeled phosphate bone imaging agent is the
A. kidneys
B. liver
C. bone marrow
D. bladder wall
E. genitals
REF: 50-p. 116

1079. The usual adult dose of ^{99m}Tc MDP used in bone scintigraphy is
A. 2-3 mCi
B. 4-6 mCi
C. 8-10 mCi
D. 15-20 mCi
E. 25-30 mCi
REF: 49-p. 209

1080. The main disadvantage of ^{99m}Tc MDP or ^{99m}Tc HMDP bone scintigraphy is the
A. associated high morbidity
B. extensive patient preparation
C. relatively low specificity of an abnormal "hot spot" finding
D. difficulty of obtaining high (> 90%) radioactive labels
E. high incidence of reported patient reactions after dose administration
REF: 50-p. 117

1081. The distribution of a ^{99m}Tc labeled phosphate agent within the skeleton of normal growing children is ____________ related.
A. age
B. weight
C. sex
D. race
E. geographically
REF: 57-p. 137

1082. High quality skeletal images may be obtained _______ after ^{99m}Tc MDP administration.
A. immediately
B. 30 minutes
C. 1 hour
D. 2 hours
E. 4 hours
REF: 50-p. 115

1083. If not contraindicated, one way to improve the quality of bone images after ^{99m}Tc MDP administration is to instruct the patient to
A. drink at least one liter of fluid
B. not eat prior to the scan
C. engage in as vigorous activity as possible
D. have a cleansing enema
E. refrain from any manual labor
REF: 54-6(10s):68, 1981

1084. The patient is requested to empty his bladder prior to bone scintigraphy to

A. reduce the radiation dose delivered to the bladder
B. prevent bladder activity from obscuring pelvic detail
C. to facilitate radionuclidic clearance from the vascular pool
D. A and B
E. B and C
F. all of the above
REF: 49-p. 211

1085. Although a rectilinear scanner may be used for whole body bone scintigraphy, it has a major drawback in that

A. spatial resolution is poor
B. too much time is required to scan the entire body
C. most systems do not allow wide enough margins to adequately image a heavy patient
D. information densities are too low with typical doses of ^{99m}Tc labeled phosphate compounds
E. the focused collimators required produce artifacts
REF: 32-p. 393

1086. When bone imaging with a large field of view gamma camera, the technologist should image all of the following views EXCEPT

A. anterior thorax
B. anterior pelvis
C. anterior abdomen
D. posterior lumbar spine
E. posterior thorax
REF: 49-p. 17

1087. A minimum number of ____________ counts is recommended to obtain technically adequate bone scintigrams accomplished on whole body imaging tables.

A. 100k
B. 500k
C. 1000k
D. 5000k
E. 10,000k
REF: 32-p. 392

1088. When a gamma scintillation camera is attached to a whole body imaging accessory device, the detector's field of view becomes
A. less sensitive to gamma radiations
B. more likely to undergo uniformity changes
C. unreliable to count rate changes
D. limited by its circular shape
E. rectangular in shape
REF: 32-p. 392

1089. Areas of increased activity noted on bone images occur from all the following pathologic conditions EXCEPT
A. metastatic tumors
B. avascular necrosis
C. fractures
D. Paget's disease
E. arthritides
REF: 50-p. 117

1090. Bone scintigraphy is used primarily for
A. locating primary bone tumors
B. locating and assessing the extent of metastatic bone lesions
C. evaluating arthritic disease
D. diagnosis of skeletal inflammatory disease
E. evaluating skeletal pain
REF: 32-p. 395

1091. Besides checking for bony metastatic disease, routine bone scintigraphy can be used for
A. therapeutic treatment of metastatic lesions by quadrupling the usual adult dose
B. selection of biopsy sites in patients having negative radiographs but positive scans
C. determining bone mineralization of menopausal females
D. bone retention studies of patients with osteomalacia
E. GFR (glomerular filtration rate) determination as an incidental finding
REF: 54-6(10s):68, 1981

1092. Metastatic lesions which appear as having normal or decreased ^{99m}Tc MDP uptake are most likely due to a primary carcinoma of

A. osteogenic sarcoma
B. multiple myeloma
C. Ewings
D. prostate
E. hepatoma
REF: 49-p. 212

1093. As a general statement, the most common site for metastatic spread of cancer is the

A. skeleton
B. lungs
C. brain
D. lymphatic system
E. liver
REF: 58-p. 555

1094. About ____________% of all metastatic lesions from breast and prostate carcinoma are localized in the axial skeleton.

A. 10
B. 20
C. 40
D. 60
E. 80
REF: 58-p. 555

1095. Metastatic lesions from primary lung carcinoma appear on bone scintigraphy as being located

A. primarily in the skull
B. primarily in the spinal column
C. exclusively in the spinal column
D. primarily in the thoracic cage
E. randomly distributed throughout the entire skeleton
REF: 58-p. 555

1096. Increased activity noted in the lower cervical spine on a whole body bone scan on an older patient is most likely due to
A. stress fracture
B. thyroid cartilage
C. thyroid organ
D. "pinched nerve"
E. degenerative changes
REF: 8-139(3):703, 1981

1097. A potential pitfall to interpreting a bone scan on the basis of symmetrical appearance is a patient with a diagnosis of
A. bilateral breast carcinoma
B. osteoporosis
C. osteosarcoma
D. arthritis
E. Paget's disease
REF: 54-6(10s):68, 1981

1098. A well-aligned series of focal "hot" spots along the rib cage noted on a bone scan is most likely due to
A. Ewings sarcoma
B. breast cancer metastatic disease
C. trauma
D. primary hyperparathyroidism
E. osteomyelitis
REF: 54-6(10s):68, 1981

1099. As a general rule, fractures become positive on bone scans at about ____________ post trauma.
A. 1-2 hours
B. 3-5 days
C. 1 week
D. 2 weeks
E. 1 month
REF: 54-6(10s):68, 1981

1100. The majority (approx. 90%) of abnormal scans of uncomplicated bone fracture sites in adults return to normal after injury by
A. 1 week
B. 1 month
C. 6 months
D. 1 year
E. 2 years
REF: 4-20:1227, 1979

1101. To rule out urinary tract obstruction as an incidental finding on a posterior whole body bone scan, the patient should
A. have a second dose of ^{99m}Tc MDP administered
B. be imaged in the anterior position
C. be injected with a dose of ^{99m}Tc DTPA
D. have an intravenous pyelogram
E. be ambulated and reimaged
REF: 47-p. 219

1102. Bone scans of patients with long-term steroid therapy typically appear as having
A. increased multiple focal areas of skeletal activity
B. multiple focal areas of decreased skeletal activity
C. generalized intense increased skeletal activity—the so called "superscan"
D. generalized decreased skeletal activity
E. no difference from a normal scan
REF: 5-12:184, 1982

1103. Bone affected with Paget's disease characteristically appears on bone scintigraphy as having
A. multifocal, significantly decreased areas of activity
B. patchy, slightly decreased areas
C. multifocal areas of slightly increased activity
D. continuous areas of intense activity uptake
E. isodense regions which can only be identified on plain radiographs
REF: 5-6:47, 1976.

1104. Decreased uptake of ^{99m}Tc MDP occurs in bones that are
A. subjected to localized fields of high irradiation
B. necrosed
C. fractured
D. A and B
E. A and C
F. B and C
REF: 50-p. 117

1105. The occurrence of bone necrosis due to infarction is best studied by the use of both 99 mTc MDP
A. ^{99m}Tc sulfur colloid
B. ^{99m}Tc PYP
C. $^{99m}TcO_4^-$
D. ^{67}Ga
E. ^{111}In red blood cells
REF: 5-6:83, 1976

1106. The so-called "superscan" of bone scintigraphy has ____________ bone uptake activity and ____________ kidneys/bladder uptake
A. marked decreased; decreased
B. marked decreased; increased
C. marked increased; increased
D. marked increased; decreased
E. normal; increased
REF: 58-p. 554

1107. Soft tissue concentration of ^{99m}Tc MDP on delayed images may occur in the
A. breast
B. lungs
C. brain
D. A and B
E. B and C
F. all of the above
REF: 56-p. 158

1108. The most common cause for findings of diffuse asymmetries in ^{99m}Tc labeled phosphate bone scans is
A. extensive neoplastic disease
B. lack of proper patient hydration
C. nonuniformity of the gamma camera
D. rotation and malpositioning of the patient
E. radiation contamination on the patient
REF: 56-p. 139

1109. A slight extravasation of ^{99m}Tc MDP during intravenous administration will cause
A. an area of markedly increased activity
B. an area of markedly decreased activity
C. no noticeable effect on an image
D. the ^{99m}Tc "tag" to break down
E. microcolloids to form and therefore visualization of the lungs
REF: 47-p. 217

1110. The "glove" phenomenon, an area of increased ^{99m}Tc MDP activity within soft tissue or bone in an extremity, is due to
A. breakdown of the MDP
B. an arterial injection of the MDP
C. MDP microcolloidal formation
D. improper patient hydration
E. regional ischemia
REF: 47-p. 219

1111. Bone scintigraphy should not be used as a diagnostic tool for osteomyelitis in a neonate until the infant is at least ____________ old.
A. 2 days
B. 1 week
C. 4-6 weeks
D. 10-12 weeks
E. 8-10 months
REF: 38-p. 59

1112. What phases of tracer activity are examined in a three-phase bone scan using ^{99m}Tc MDP?
A. Concentrating, blood pool, and osseous
B. Concentrating, vascular, and blood pool
C. Vascular, blood pool, and excretory
D. Vascular, osseous, and excretory
E. Vascular, blood pool, and osseous
REF: 53-p. 210

1113. Three-phase bone scintigraphy is best used to distinguish
A. cellulitis from osteomyelitis
B. osteonecrosis from osteoporosis
C. Paget's disease from osteonecrosis
D. primary tumors from metastatic tumors
E. recent fractures from metastatic tumors
REF: 49-p. 213

1114. Quantitative digital bone imaging has been most helpful in the diagnosis of
A. osteomyelitis
B. sacroiliitis
C. Paget's disease
D. osteoporosis
E. Ewings sarcoma
REF: 58-p. 571

1115. Radionuclidic joint scintigraphy is performed using
A. $^{99m}TcO_4^-$
B. ^{99m}Tc MDP
C. ^{99m}Tc DTPA
D. A and B
E. A and C
F. B and C
REF: 58-p. 569

1116. ^{99m}Tc phosphate retention studies accomplished on whole body counters are used to measure
A. the extent of bony metastatic involvement
B. the degree of skeletal metabolism
C. the clearance function of the kidneys
D. the potential of high risk patients to develop infections
E. the effects of arthritis
REF: 56-p. 158

17. PULMONARY

DIRECTIONS: Each of the questions or incomplete statements below is followed by a list of suggested answers or completions. Select the **one** that is **BEST** in each case.

1117. The lungs' main function is the
 A. movement and exchange of gases
 B. moderation of water loss
 C. regulation of body enzymes
 D. conversion of ATP to ADP
 E. destruction of harmful gases in the body
 REF: 22-p. 119

1118. The trachea divides into the
 A. alveolar ducts
 B. alveolar sacs
 C. lobar bronchi
 D. main stem bronchi
 E. respiratory bronchioles
 REF: 32-p. 272

1119. The lobes of the lungs are anatomically further divided into sections known as
A. lobular divisions
B. segments
C. subsegments
D. functional units
E. lobar planes
REF: 47-p. 141

1120. The primary respiratory muscles are the
A. intercostal and diaphragm
B. intercostal and abdominal
C. abdominal and thoracic
D. abdominal and diaphragm
E. thoracic and abdominal
REF: 22-p. 120

1121. The approximate lung blood supply ratio of the right and left pulmonary arteries to systemic circulation is about
A. 1:1
B. 2:1
C. 4:1
D. 7:1
E. 9:1
REF: 1-p. 505

1122. The exchange of respiratory gases occurs at the alveoli. Each alveolus is in contact with
A. the bronchi
B. a bronchiole
C. a capillary
D. muscle cells
E. lymphatic tissue
REF: 22-p. 119

1123. Most of the resistance to air flow in the lungs is found at the
A. alveolar sacs
B. alveolar ducts
C. respiratory bronchioles
D. terminal bronchioles
E. lobar bronchi
REF: 32-p. 272

1124. The "tidal volume" is defined as the volume of air within the lungs

A. delivered after a maximal inspiration
B. delivered after a maximal expiration
C. of one resting normal breath
D. at the end of a quiet expiration
E. at full inspiration
REF: 1-p. 506

1125. Normal human lungs in the upright position have ____________ ventilation per unit lung volume from the apices of the lungs to the bases.

A. a 1.5 to 2.0 increase in
B. a 4.0 to 5.5 increase in
C. a 1.5 to 2.0 decrease in
D. a 4.0 to 5.5 decrease in
E. approximately the same
REF: 56-p. 51

1126. Typical preparations of ^{99m}Tc MAA have average particle sizes ranging from

A. 0.1 μm–0.4 μm
B. 0.1 μm–1.4 μm
C. 10 μm–14 μm
D. 10 μm–40 μm
E. 40 μm–100 μm
REF: 5-10:199, 1980

1127. An average ^{99m}Tc MAA pulmonary dose consisting of particles with a mean size of 30 μm in a healthy patient blocks almost no lung capillaries but about ____________% of precapillary arterioles.

A. 0.1
B. 1.0
C. 5.0
D. 10.0
E. 15.0
REF: 33-p. 41

1128. The ideal number of ^{99m}Tc MAA particles for lung perfusion scintigraphy in adults images from

A. 15,000-60,000
B. 60,000-250,000
C. 60,000-1,000,000
D. 250,000-1,000,000
E. 1,000,000-6,000,000
REF: 3-10(4):225, 1982

1129. The recommended number of particles in a dose of ^{99m}Tc MAA or ^{99m}Tc HAM for a newborn should be limited to

A. 5000
B. 50,000
C. 150,000
D. 250,000
E. 500,000
REF: 3-10(4):226, 1982

1130. The localization mechanism of either ^{99m}Tc MAA or ^{99m}Tc HAM within the lungs is by

A. mechanical blockage
B. sequestration
C. phagocytosis
D. pinocytosis
E. active transport
REF: 33-p. 40

1131. The average biological half life for ^{99m}Tc labeled macroaggregated albumin is on the order of

A. 30-60 minutes
B. 1-2 hours
C. 4-6 hours
D. 10-12 hours
E. 1-2 days
REF: 33-p. 40

1132. The advantage of using ^{99m}Tc human albumin microspheres (HAM) over ^{99m}Tc macroaggregated albumin (MAA) is that the ^{99m}Tc HAM

A. is cleared more quickly from the lungs
B. is less costly
C. has a lower incidence of adverse reactions
D. has a more uniform particle
E. delivers a significantly lower radiation dose to the patient

REF: 54-p. 150

1133. It has been shown experimentally that the toxicity of particulate lung radiopharmaceuticals is essentially the result of

A. the number of particles injected
B. the size of the particles injected
C. the total radiation dose to the lungs
D. A and B
E. B and C
F. all of the above

REF: 4-19:1204, 1978

1134. ^{99m}Tc MAA is usually injected into a supine patient as this position

A. prevents the particles from entering systemic circulation
B. is less likely to form microembolisms
C. allows more even distribution of particles from the lung apex to the base
D. matches the ventilation and perfusion patterns of lungs more evenly
E. removes the particles from circulation more quickly and efficiently

REF: 1-p. 509

1135. After injection of ^{99m}Tc MAA or ^{99m}Tc HAM, perfusion imaging may be started within

A. 1–2 minutes
B. 10–15 minutes
C. 20–30 minutes
D. 45–60 minutes
E. 90–120 minutes

REF: 50-p. 197

1136. If a syringe of ^{99m}Tc MAA containing either a non-uniform mixture or blood clots (from aspirated blood) is injected into a patient

A. the ^{99m}Tc MAA will be shunted to systemic circulation
B. the ^{99m}Tc "tag" spots will appear on the images MAA
C. multiple focal "hot" spots will appear on the images
D. 60-80% of the dose will adhere to the sides of the syringe
E. activity uptake in the liver and spleen will be noted
REF: 1-p. 509

1137. The most sensitive screening tool for the diagnosis of pulmonary embolism is

A. the chest x-ray
B. clinical symptoms
C. ventilation/perfusion scintigraphy
D. chemical serum enzyme studies
E. pulmonary arteriography
REF: 1-p. 511

1138. The major cause of pulmonary embolization is

A. blunt trauma injury
B. fatty emboli from arteriosclerosis
C. tumor emboli formed within the lungs
D. air embolism from faulty intravenous infusion
E. thrombi from deep venous thrombophlebitis
REF: 1-p. 511

1139. In addition to a ^{99m}Tc MAA perfusion scan to properly diagnose pulmonary embolism a (an) __________ must be performed on the patient.

A. electrocardiogram
B. plain chest film
C. xenon ventilation scan
D. A and B
E. B and C
F. all of the above
REF: 5-10:198, 1980

1140. A segmental or lobar perfusion defect seen on ^{99m}Tc MAA perfusion scintigraphy without the benefit of a ventilation scan is ____________ in the diagnosis of pulmonary embolism.
A. both sensitive and specific
B. sensitive but nonspecific
C. not sensitive but specific
D. not sensitive and nonspecific
E. uninterpretable
REF: 38-p. 127

1141. ^{99m}Tc MAA lung perfusion defects due to acute pulmonary embolism characteristically are
A. larger (lobar or polysegmental)
B. associated with a normal ventilation study
C. apt to change with time
D. A and B
E. B and C
F. all of the above
REF: 58-p. 45

1142. A perfusion lung scan may detect the effects of an embolism as small as
A. 1 mm
B. 5 mm
C. 3 cm
D. 8 cm
E. 10 cm
REF: 38-p. 127

1143. To remove any doubt on the diagnosis of pulmonary embolism versus chronic obstructive lung disease on an abnormal lung perfusion scan, imaging should be repeated at
A. 2–3 hours
B. 10–12 hours
C. 1–2 days
D. 3–4 days
E. 5–7 days
REF: 33-p. 51

1144. Perfusion imaging of a patient accomplished in the upright position permits
A. better lung base visualization
B. a decrease in the cardiac silhouette
C. fewer required images
D. a longer biologic half-life of the particles
E. noninterference of kidney shine through
REF: 5-10:200, 1980

1145. Besides the anterior and posterior views, other recommended projections for perfusion imaging include the left and right
A. anterior obliques
B. posterior obliques
C. laterals
D. A and B
E. B and C
F. all of the above
REF: 50-p. 198

1146. A perfusion scan accomplished on a patient with known emphysema is characterized by
A. an increase in the size of the lungs
B. an increase in the size of the aortic arch silhouette
C. visualization of the bases of the lung on the anterior image
D. a decrease in the size of the lungs
E. a decrease in the size of the aortic arch
REF: 36-p. 462

1147. Besides being useful in the diagnosis and management of patients with pulmonary embolism, ventilation/perfusion scintigraphy is also useful in the management of patients with
A. carcinoma of the bronchus
B. respiratory tract infections
C. diseases of the pleura
D. interstitial lung diseases
E. chronic air flow obstruction
REF: 56-p. 41

1148. The most common finding of bronchogenic carcinoma on a ^{99m}Tc MAA perfusion scan is

A. uniform increased activity in one lung
B. multiple focal areas of increased activity
C. complete absence of activity in one lung
D. multiple focal areas of decreased activity in both lungs
E. patchy decreased activity in both lungs
REF: 1-p. 514

1149. The "fissure sign" (decreased interlobar activity) when observed on radionuclide pulmonary perfusion images is most likely due to

A. bronchogenic carcinoma
B. pulmonary embolism
C. chronic obstructive pulmonary disease
D. pleural effusion
E. acute asthmatic attack
REF: 33-p. 53

1150. The physical half-life of ^{133}Xe is ____________ and its biologic half-life is __________.

A. 72 hours; < 30 seconds
B. 72 hours; 1 hour
C. 5.2 days; < 30 seconds
D. 5.2 days; 1 hour
E. 5.3 days; 7.2 hours
REF: 53-p. 151

1151. A proper ^{133}Xe ventilation study should include

A. a first breath image
B. equilibrium images
C. multiple washout images
D. A and B
E. B and C
F. all of the above
REF: 42-p. 114

1152. The major factor that determines the distribution of ^{133}Xe in a normal patient is
A. lung volume
B. patient positioning
C. perfusion patency
D. inhalation rate
E. local compliance
REF: 53-p. 151

1153. The agent(s) used for lung ventilation studies that does (do) not enable the accomplishment of washout studies is (are)
A. ^{127}Xe
B. ^{133}Xe
C. ^{81m}Kr
D. A and B
E. A and C
F. B and C
REF: 54-p. 152

1154. All of the following are advantages of using ^{127}Xe over ^{133}Xe for ventilation studies EXCEPT ^{127}Xe
A. allows perfusion scintigraphy to be performed before the ventilation study
B. delivers less of a radiation dose to the patient
C. is less costly per mCi
D. has decreased absorption in soft tissue
E. has better storage capabilities due to its longer half-life
REF: 53-p. 152

1155. A ^{133}Xe ventilation pattern of an inhomogeneous washin, a patchy but more uniform equilibrium, and delayed washout of trapped areas of the gas are all characteristic of
A. congestive heart failure
B. bronchogenic carcinoma
C. pulmonary embolism
D. chronic obstructive pulmonary disease
E. pneumonia
REF: 33-p. 56

1156. The most prevalent reason for ^{133}Xe localization and retention in the liver during a ventilation equilibrium and washout study is
A. hepatic contusion
B. hepatitis
C. liver fatty infiltrates
D. Hodgkin's lymphoma
E. vena cava obstruction
REF: 4-20(5):397, 1979

1157. All of the following are true statements about the use of ^{99m}Tc MAA for perfusion scrintigraphy and ^{133}Xe for ventilation scintigraphy EXCEPT
A. the energy of ^{99m}Tc is better suited for a gamma camera
B. ^{133}Xe ventilation can usually be done in only one projection, while multiple projections of ^{99m}Tc perfusion are easily obtained
C. less patient cooperation is required for the ventilation study
D. the ventilation study is best performed before the perfusion study
E. both the ventilation and perfusion study can be accomplished on comatose patients
REF: 38-p. 130

1158. Most of the difficulties associated with aerosols for ventilation imaging are related to
A. patient compliance
B. the variation in particle size
C. the excessive cost of required equipment
D. potential dangerous side effects
E. the invasiveness of the procedure
REF: 56-p. 74

1159. A ^{99m}Tc DTPA aerosol study may be performed after ^{99m}Tc MAA perfusion if

A. thc perfusion study is normal
B. the patient is mechanically ventilated
C. the patient can hold his breath for long periods of time
D. a narrow gamma camera PHA "window" is used
E. three to five times as much ^{99m}Tc DTPA is used
REF: 56-p. 75

1160. ^{99m}Tc DTPA aerosol images have the advantage(s) over ^{133}Xe ventilation images of being

A. better suited for gamma camera imaging
B. more sensitive for detection of air flow obstruction
C. able to be accomplished immediately following the perfusion study
D. A and B
E. A and C
F. all of the above
REF: 56-p. 75

1161. Bronchial arterial circulation may be best assessed with a dynamic scintigraphy study using

A. $^{99m}TcO_4^-$
B. ^{67}Ga
C. ^{99m}Tc HAM
D. ^{131}I MAA
E. ^{99m}Tc MAA
REF: 38-p. 129

1162. Acute bacterial pneumonia appears on ventilation/perfusion images as areas of

A. slightly decreased perfusion and slightly decreased ventilation
B. slightly decreased perfusion and markedly decreased ventilation
C. slightly increased perfusion and slightly decreased ventilation
D. slightly increased perfusion and markedly increased ventilation
E. markedly increased perfusion and markedly increased ventilation
REF: 58-p. 483

1163. The best radiopharmaceutical which actively concentrates within pulmonary tumor is
A. ^{99m}Tc MAA
B. ^{67}Ga
C. ^{99m}Tc MDP
D. ^{133}Xe
E. ^{127}Xe
REF: 58-p. 467

18. GASTROINTESTINAL TRACT

DIRECTIONS: Each of the questions or incomplete statements below is followed by a list of suggested answers or completions. Select the **one** that is **BEST** in each case.

1164. One indication for doing a GI protein loss determination is

A. gastric carcinoma
B. biliary obstruction
C. aplastic anemia
D. malabsorption syndrome
E. acute gastritis
REF: 36-p. 292

1165. The best radionuclide and carrier for determining GI protein loss is

A. ^{99m}Tc - albumin
B. ^{51}Cr - albumin
C. ^{131}In- albumin
D. ^{131}I - albumin
E. ^{125}I - albumin
REF: 18-p. 154

1166. A positive diagnosis of protein loss using ^{51}Cr - albumin is made in 96 hours when

A. urinary excretion is more than 5% of the administered dose
B. ^{51}Cr is retained in the stomach for less than 1 hour
C. ^{51}Cr blood levels exceed 10% of the administered dose
D. fecal excretion is more than 1% of the administered dose
E. saliva samples exceed 10% of the administered dose

REF: 36-p. 293

1167. The incidence of salivary gland tumors ____________ with the gland's size; tumor malignancy ____________ with decreasing gland size.

A. increases; increases
B. increases; decreases
C. increases; remains the same
D. decreases; decreases
E. decreases; increases
F. decreases; remains the same

REF: 5-11(4):259, 1981

1168. Physiologic information that can be ascertained by $^{99m}TcO_4^-$ salivary scrintigraphy includes alterations in the gland's usual

A. perfusion
B. trapping mechanism
C. excretory function
D. A and B
E. B and C
F. all of the above

REF: 5-11(4):259, 1981

1169. The patient's head should be placed in the __________ position against the gamma camera for the dynamic position of $^{99m}TcO_4^-$ salivary scrintigraphy.

A. posterior
B. lateral
C. vertex
D. Towne's
E. Water's

REF: 36-p. 566

1170. During salivary gland scintigraphy a dose of perchlorate or a few drops of lemon juice is given to the patient to

A. quicken the concentration $^{99m}TcO_4^-$ in the glands
B. speed up imaging time by causing the salivary glands to quickly excrete the $^{99m}TcO_4^-$
C. block $^{99m}TcO_4^-$ uptake of the thyroid gland and choroid plexus
D. decrease the uptake of $^{99m}TcO_4^-$ in the sublingual glands thereby maximizing uptake in the parotid glands
E. increase the perfusion and therefore the concentration of $^{99m}TcO_4^-$ in the glands
REF: 5-11(4):259, 1981

1171. The main problem associated with $^{99m}TcO_4^-$ salivary gland scintigraphy is the fact that it is not

A. useful to evaluate the physiology of the glands
B. very specific
C. very sensitive
D. helpful in evaluating unilateral disease
E. a relatively easy procedure to perform
REF: 50-p. 144

1172. In ^{99m}Tc sulfur colloid gastroesophageal reflux scintigraphy, the radioactivity is delivered to the patient

A. as a liquid meal
B. as a solid meal
C. slowly, intramuscularly
D. as a bolus intravenously
E. in a volume of less than .25 ml
REF: 47-p. 211

1173. Gastroesophageal reflux scintigraphy is considered positive when

A. activity "hangs up" in the stomach
B. the esophagus fails to visualize within 1 hour after radionuclide administration
C. the small bowel is visualized
D. patchy "cold" areas appear in the stomach
E. any activity is visualized in the esophagus
REF: 32-p. 339

1174. Fifteen minutes following the oral administration of 300 ml orange juice containing ^{99m}Tc sulfur colloid, a patient's esophagus is visualized. If the activity persists after the patient drank 30 ml of water, the most likely cause would be

A. hiatal hernia
B. esophageal motility disorder
C. esophageal reflux
D. chronic esophagitis
E. chronic gastritis
REF: 14-p. 104

1175. The radionuclidic procedure for determining gastric half time emptying of the stomach requires the patient to be

A. fasting 6 hours prior to scanning
B. predosed with Lugol's solution
C. previously intravenously injected with 10 mg pentagastrin
D. examined by an upper GI barium study just prior to the nuclear scan
E. cooperative due to the lumbar puncture for radionuclide administration
REF: 36-p. 572

1176. Besides requiring a gamma camera, gastric emptying half time is determined using a ^{99m}Tc sulfur colloid labeled food marker and a (an)

A. well counter
B. multiprobe counting system
C. data storage device or a computer
D. physiologic synchronizer
E. ionization chamber
REF: 36-p. 572

1177. The best "tag" of ^{99m}Tc sulfur colloid to a solid food marker for the determination of gastric emptying time is accomplished with

A. cooked egg whites
B. chicken liver
C. hamburger
D. beef stew
E. lasagna
REF: 14-p. 92

1178. The best radiopharmaceutical used to localize the pancreas along with ^{99m}Tc sulfur colloid to aid in positioning is
A. ^{75}Selenomethionine
B. ^{67}Gallium citrate
C. ^{201}Thallium chloride
D. ^{111}Indium leukocytes
E. ^{18}Florine
REF: 49-p. 37

1179. The usual adult dose of ^{75}Selenomethionine for pancreas imaging is
A. 250 mCi
B. 500 mCi
C. 1.0 mCi
D. 5.0 mCi
E. 10 mCi
REF: 32-p. 337

1180. A Meckel's diverticulum is a congenital outpouching containing ectopic gastric mucosa usually located within the distal 100 cm of the
A. jejunum
B. descending colon
C. ileum
D. duodenum
E. transverse colon
REF: 4-22(8):732, 1981

1181. Meckel's diverticula occur in approximately ________% of the general population.
A. 1-3
B. 5-10
C. 15-20
D. 30-40
E. 50-60
REF: 4-22(7):647, 1981

1182. The usual imaging protocol for Meckel's diverticulum scintigraphy calls for acquiring 500k anterior images of the abdomen every ___________ up to _________ after $^{99m}TcO_4^-$ is administered.

A. 1-2 minutes; 30 minutes
B. 5-10 minutes; 60 minutes
C. 15-20 minutes; 90 minutes
D. 30 minutes; 4 hours
E. hour; 6 hours
REF: 36-p. 571

1183. A positive finding on a Meckel's diverticulum scan appears as a

A. focal "hot" area
B. focal "cold" area
C. patchy diffuse "hot" area
D. patchy diffuse "cold" area
E. either a "hot" or "cold" patchy diffuse area
REF: 14-p. 145

1184. A dose of ___________ helps concentrate $^{99m}TcO_4^-$ in a Meckel's diverticulum containing ectopic gastric mucosa.

A. pentagastrin
B. atropine
C. secretin
D. perchlorate
E. aluminum hydroxide
REF: 4-22(7):647, 1981

1185. The presence of Barrett's esophagus, an abnormality of the esophagus which contains ectopic gastric mucosa, may be determined by scintigraphic means using

A. ^{99m}Tc sulfur colloid
B. ^{99m}Tc DTPA
C. $^{99m}TcO_4^-$
D. ^{99m}Tc HSA
E. ^{99m}Tc GHA
REF: 4-22(8):735, 1981

1186. The most definitive and sensitive tool available to clinicians to detect active lower gastrointestinal bleeds on an emergency basis is (the)

A. radionuclide procedure
B. barium enema
C. colonoscopy
D. thorough patient's history
E. CAT scan
REF: 14-p. 122

1187. Intraabdominal bleeds are best detected by imaging methods using

A. ^{51}Cr labeled RBCS
B. ^{99m}Tc labeled RBCs
C. ^{99m}Tc labeled human serum albumin (HSA)
D. ^{131}I labeled HSA
E. ^{99m}Tc labeled macroaggregated albumin (MAA)
REF: 14-p. 127

1188. All of the following have been cited as disadvantages of the use of ^{99m}Tc red blood cells (RBCs) over ^{99m}Tc sulfur colloid (S.C.) for the red detection of acute gastrointestinal bleeding EXCEPT

A. blood flow must be greater with the use of ^{99m}Tc RBCs than with ^{99m}Tc S.C. for initial detection of the site
B. a degree of location uncertainty exists with delayed imaging of ^{99m}Tc RBCs due to possible bowel transit but does not with ^{99m}Tc S.C.
C. nasal suction or tedious labeling procedures must be performed with ^{99m}Tc RBCs to avoid the presence of free pertechnetate which may mimic a bleed but not with ^{99m}Tc S.C.
D. upper gastrointestinal bleeds are not detectable with ^{99m}Tc RBCs but may be with ^{99m}Tc S.C.
E. the inconvenience of imaging over 24 hours with ^{99m}Tc RBCs versus the relatively short protocol required for ^{99m}Tc S.C.
REF: 47-p. 201

1189. One shortcoming of the use of ^{99m}Tc sulfur colloid for site detection of acute gastrointestinal bleeding is that

A. the patient must have been kept NPO at least 6 hours before the procedure begins
B. bleeding flow rates greater than 5.0 ml/min must be present for localization
C. the patient must be bleeding at the time of injection in order for the bleed to be detected
D. sulfur colloid may aggravate the bleed
E. computer-enhanced images are required for interpretation
REF: 38-p. 45

1190. The localization mechanism of ^{99m}Tc sulfur colloid at the site of an active gastrointestinal bleed is

A. active transport
B. vascular extravasation
C. capillary blockage
D. simple diffusion
E. RBC binding
REF: 14-p. 128

1191. Experimental data have shown that gastrointestinal bleeds may be detected with the use of ^{99m}Tc sulfur colloid with bleeding rates as low as

A. 0.01 ml/min
B. 0.1 ml/min
C. 1.0 ml/min
D. 10.0 ml/min
E. 100.0 ml/min
REF: 8-124:753, 1971

1192. A typical protocol for GI bleed scintigraphy with ^{99m}Tc sulfur colloid requires anterior abdomen images to be acquired on a large field of view camera every ____________ minutes up to ____________.

A. 1–2; 15 minutes
B. 5; 15 minutes
C. 15; 1 hour
D. 15; 3 hours
E. 30; 3 hours
REF: 47-p. 202

1193. The kinetic model of hepatobiliary tracers can be described by the competition of radiopharmaceutical clearance between the liver and the
A. soft tissue
B. muscle
C. lungs
D. spleen
E. kidneys
REF: 15-p. 24

1194. The largest estimated radiation absorbed dose from a ^{99m}Tc IDA analog administration in a normally hepatic functioning patient is delivered to the
A. liver
B. gallbladder
C. large bowel
D. kidneys
E. ovaries/testes
REF: 14-p. 52

1195. The ^{99m}Tc labeled hepatobiliary agents are used for all of the following purposes EXCEPT
A. determination of metastatic liver disease
B. disclosure of bile leak
C. assessment of cystic duct patency
D. assessment of altered cholangiointestine anatomy
E. determination of hepatocellular function by the rate of activity accumulation
REF: 36-p. 519

1196. The major cause of focal biliary obstruction in a neonate is
A. cystic dilation of the common bile duct
B. hepatic fibrosis
C. hepatic infarction
D. acute cholecystitis
E. biliary atresia
REF: 15-p. 39

1197. The usual adult dose of ^{99m}Tc labeled hepatobiliary agents is
- **A.** 200-250 mCi
- **B.** 0.5-1.0 mCi
- **C.** 3.0 mCi
- **D.** 5.0 mCi
- **E.** 10.0 mCi

REF: 32-p. 333

1198. The patient preparation for ^{99m}Tc IDA scrintigraphy to evaluate cystic duct patency is
- **A.** NPO orders for at least 2 hours prior to the study
- **B.** a cleansing enema completed just before radiopharmaceutical administration
- **C.** a fatty meal at the time of beginning the study
- **D.** a dose of pentagastrin prior to radiopharmaceutical administration
- **E.** complete hydration

REF: 36-p. 519

1199. To evaluate hepatocyte function with ^{99m}Tc labeled hepatobiliary agents, imaging must begin __________ after administration of the radiopharmaceutical.
- **A.** immediately
- **B.** 30 minutes
- **C.** 1 hour
- **D.** 2 hours
- **E.** 4 hours

REF: 49-p. 57

1200. Two hours after administration to a normal patient, most of the ^{99m}Tc HIDA should be located in the
- **A.** liver
- **B.** gut
- **C.** kidneys
- **D.** bladder
- **E.** gallbladder

REF: 15-p. 26

1201. Visualization of the gallbladder within 20 minutes after the injection of ^{99m}Tc DISIDA implies
A. acute cholecystitis
B. a patent cystic duct
C. partial to full hepatic vein obstruction
D. a breakdown of the radiopharmaceutical
E. an obstructed bile duct
REF: 14-p. 56

1202. If the gallbladder common bile duct and the duodenum are not visualized within 1 hour on ^{99m}Tc IDA hepatobiliary images, delayed imaging should be accomplished hourly up to
A. 2 hours
B. 4 hours
C. 12 hours
D. 1 day
E. 2 days
REF: 47-p. 205

1203. A reliable sign of chronic cholecystitis in patients with recent symptoms from ^{99m}Tc IDA analog scintigraphy is
A. 15 minute gallbladder visualization but with no gut visualization
B. 15 minute gallbladder visualization but with delayed (> 1 hour) gut visualization
C. 15 minute gallbladder visualization and gut visualization within 30 minutes
D. delayed (> 1 hour) gallbladder visualization but no gut visualization
E. delayed (> 1 hour) gallbladder visualization but gut visualization within 30 minutes
REF: 14-p. 56

1204. Hepatic uptake and gut excretion of ^{99m}Tc IDA analogs without gallbladder visualization at 4 hours is indicative of
A. acute cholecystitis
B. chronic cholecystitis
C. biliary atresia
D. a nonpatent common duct
E. a patent cystic duct
REF: 47-p. 206

1205. A dose of ____________ followed by a second dose of ^{99m}Tc IDA may allow a previously nonvisualized gall-bladder to accumulate activity.
A. pentagastrin
B. lasix
C. cholecystokinin
D. cimetidine
E. atropine
REF: 14-p. 53

19. CARDIOVASCULAR SYSTEM

DIRECTIONS: Each of the questions or incomplete statements below is followed by a list of suggested answers or completions. Select the **one** that is **BEST** in each case.

1206. The heart wall is composed of ____________ tissue layers.
A. 2
B. 3
C. 4
D. 5
E. 6
REF: 16-p. 468

1207. The membranous sac which surrounds the heart is called the
A. auricle
B. endocardium
C. myocardium
D. vortex
E. pericardium
REF: 16-p. 457

1208. The portion of the heart wall separating the right and left ventricle is the
A. apex
B. septum
C. base
D. endocardium
E. epicardium
REF: 16–p. 467

1209. The ____________ of the heart is (are) responsible for receiving systemic venous blood and pumping it into the pulmonary circulation for oxygenation.
A. atria
B. apex
C. ventricles
D. left side
E. right side
REF: 16–p. 455

1210. The tricuspid valve in the heart is located between the
A. right atrium and right ventricle
B. right atrium and left atrium
C. left ventricle and aorta
D. left atrium and left ventricle
E. right ventricle and pulmonary artery
REF: 16–p. 463

1211. The venous blood supply returning via the superior and inferior vena cava enters the heart at the
A. right atrium
B. right ventricle
C. left ventricle
D. left coronary artery
E. left atrium
REF: 22–p. 105

1212. The pulmonary artery conveys blood from the
A. left side of the heart to the viscera
B. left side of the heart to the lungs
C. left side to the right side of the heart
D. right side of the heart to the lungs
E. right side of the heart to the viscera
REF: 16–p. 475

1213. The coronary arteries originate at the
A. ascending aorta
B. pulmonary artery
C. left pulmonary vein
D. left carotid artery
E. left subclavian vein
REF: 16-p. 476

1214. The volume of blood pumped out by the adult heart per minute is
A. 1-2 liters
B. 2-3 liters
C. 3-4 liters
D. 4-5 liters
E. 5-6 liters
REF: 22-p. 111

1215. The organ(s) receiving the greatest portion of the cardiac output under rest conditions is (are) the
A. liver and gut
B. kidneys
C. heart
D. spleen and pancreas
E. muscle
REF: 22-p. 111

1216. At rest, the normal coronary blood flow is approximately
A. 10 ml/min
B. 25 ml/min
C. 100 ml/min
D. 225 ml/min
E. 350 ml/min
REF: 47-p. 105

1217. The electrical impulse generated in the heart originates at the
A. AV (atrioventricular) node
B. SA (sinoatrial) node
C. bundle branches
D. Purkinje fiber
E. bundle of His
REF: 22-p. 107

1218. The contraction phase of the heart is called
A. systole
B. diastole
C. stroke volume
D. cardiac output
E. stroke output
REF: 32-p. 295

1219. The electrocardiogram presents a visible record of thc heart's
A. output
B. left ventricular ejection fraction
C. coronary artery perfusion
D. electrical activity
E. contraction
REF: 21-p. 4

1220. The largest deflection in a normal ECG is the
A. P wave
B. Q wave
C. R wave
D. S wave
E. T wave
REF: 21-p. 8

1221. The QRS complex in a normal ECG represents transmission of an electrical pulse through the
A. right ventricle
B. right and left ventricle
C. right atrium
D. right and left atria
E. atria and ventricles
REF: 21-p. 5

1222. In a standard 12-lead electrocardiogram precordial lead V4 is positioned on the chest at the same level as
A. V1
B. V2
C. V3
D. V5
REF: 20-p. 2

1223. Which is the only lead positioned to the right of a patient's sternum in a standard electrocardiogram?
A. AVL
B. AVF
C. V1
D. V2
E. V3
REF: 20-p. 2

1224. Which of the following is the proper number and type of leads used for a routine 12-lead electrocardiogram?
A. 2 standard limb; 4 aV 6V
B. 2 standard limb; 6 aV 4V
C. 3 standard limb; 3 aV 6V
D. 3 standard limb; 6 aV 3V
E. 6 standard limb; 2 aV 4V
REF: 20-p. 7

1225. A technical consideration essential for performing an artifact-free ECG tracing is the
A. use of electrode jelly
B. effective contact between electrode and skin
C. use of silver content electrodes
D. free, unsecured movement of electrode leads from the patient
E. upright positioning of the patient
REF: 20-p. 8

1226. The radiopharmaceutical most commonly used for the detection of acute myocardial infarction is
A. ^{99m}Tc pyrophosphate
B. ^{99m}Tc tetracycline
C. ^{99m}Tc human serum albumin
D. ^{99m}Tc microspheres
E. ^{201}Tl chloride
REF: 43-p. 258

1227. Myocardial uptake of ^{99m}Tc pyrophosphate used in acute myocardial infarct scintigraphy depends upon

A. tissue damage
B. calcification
C. blood flow
D. A and B
E. B and C
F. all of the above
REF: 43-p. 258

1228. The radiopharmaceutical with the highest acute myocardial infarct-to-normal uptake ratio is

A. ^{99m}Tc oxytetracycline
B. ^{99m}Tc diphosphonate
C. ^{99m}Tc pyrophosphate
D. ^{99m}Tc glucoheptonate
E. ^{99m}Tc tetracycline
REF: 43-p. 261

1229. The standard adult dose of ^{99m}Tc pyrophosphate used for acute myocardial infarct scintigraphy is

A. 150 uCi
B. 500 uCi
C. 5 mCi
D. 10 mCi
E. 15 mCi
REF: 43-p. 266

1230. ^{99m}Tc pyrophosphate scintigraphy for acute myocardial infarction is most sensitive in patients with

A. nonspecific ST segment changes
B. nonspecific T wave abnormalities
C. subendocardial infarction
D. transmural infarction
E. cardiomyopathy
REF: 44-p. 297

1231. Patients with acute myocardial infarction show peak ^{99m}Tc pyrophosphate uptake between ____________ after onset of symptoms.
A. 1-2 hours
B. 3-4 hours
C. 2-3 days
D. 6-7 days
E. 1-2 weeks
REF: 44-p. 299

1232. In addition to one or more left anterior obliques, the usual patient positioning for ^{99m}Tc pyrophosphate scintigraphy for acute myocardial infarction accomplished on a gamma camera includes the ____________ images.
A. left and right lateral
B. left lateral and anterior
C. right lateral and anterior
D. anterior and right anterior oblique
E. right lateral and right anterior oblique
REF: 45-p. 164

1233. An acute myocardial infarction will be detected using 201 thallium ____________ after the infarction.
A. immediately
B. 6 hours
C. 2-3 days
D. 6-7 days
E. 1-2 weeks
REF: 46-p. 167

1234. On a positive ^{99m}Tc pyrophosphate scan, to distinguish an old scar from acute myocardial infarction one should
A. double the ^{99m}Tc PYP dose
B. obtain a 12-lead electrocardiogram
C. repeat the scan at a week after first onset of symptoms
D. obtain right lateral and right anterior oblique images
E. assure that the radiopharmaceutical has no more than 5% free $^{99m}TcO_4^-$
REF: 45-p. 161

1235. The usual number of counts obtained on a left anterior oblique image as part of a ^{99m}Tc pyrophosphate acute myocardial infarct study accomplished on a standard field of view gamma camera is

A. 50,000-100,000
B. 200,000-300,000
C. 300,000-500,000
D. 500,000-700,000
E. 800,000-1,000,000
REF: 43-p. 267

1236. A positive ^{99m}Tc pyrophosphate scan for acute myocardial infarction appears as a

A. focal "hot" area
B. diffuse "hot" area
C. focal "cold" area
D. diffuse "cold" area
E. patchy "hot" or "cold" area
REF: 44-p. 300

1237. Routine imaging of ^{99m}Tc pyrophosphate for acute myocardial infarction usually is accomplished _______ after injection.

A. immediately
B. 30-60 minutes
C. 1-2 hours
D. 3-4 hours
E. 6-8 hours
REF: 44-p. 294

1238. Imaging at ____________ hours after injection of ^{99m}Tc pyrophosphate for acute myocardial infarction imaging increases the chances for a false-positive study.

A. less than 2
B. less than 4
C. more than 4
D. more than 5
E. more than 6
REF: 48-p. 35

1239. First pass radiocardiography studies using a multi-crystal gamma camera provide all of the following EXCEPT

A. qualitative anatomic information
B. diagnostic information from stress-induced studies
C. left ventricular ejection fraction
D. left ventricular time activity curves
E. reproducible ejection fractions on every heart beat
REF: 44-p. 272

1240. The usual injection site for first pass radionuclide angiocardiography is the (a)

A. carotid artery
B. circumflex coronary artery
C. basilic vein
D. hepatic vein
E. femoral vein
REF: 47-p. 128

1241. If repeat first pass radionuclide angiography studies are not contemplated, all of the following radiopharmaceuticals can be used EXCEPT

A. $^{99m}TcO_4^-$
B. ^{99m}Tc macroaggregates
C. ^{99m}Tc PYP
D. ^{99m}Tc DTPA
E. ^{99m}Tc human serum albumin
REF: 45-p. 187

1242. When repeat serial first pass angiography studies are to be performed, the radiopharmaceutical of choice is

A. $^{99m}TcO_4^-$
B. ^{99m}Tc macroaggregates
C. ^{99m}Tc PYP
D. ^{99m}Tc DTPA
E. ^{99m}Tc human serum albumin
REF: 45-p. 187

1243. The collection of data in cardiac first pass studies begins when the bolus of activity

A. is injected
B. enters the right ventricle
C. enters the pulmonary veins
D. exits from the lungs
E. exits from the left ventricle
REF: 47-p. 129

1244. The major disadvantage of using a nonimaging single crystal probe instead of a single crystal scintillation gamma for first pass cardiac studies is the probe's

A. lower counting sensitivity
B. lack of regional left ventricular function assessment capability
C. higher initial cost
D. requirement for increased patient doses
E. large physical size and storage requirements
REF: 45-p. 206

1245. The main advantage of using a multicrystal scintillation camera over a single crystal scintillation camera when performing first pass radionuclide angiography studies is that the former has better

A. spatial resolution
B. count rate capability
C. energy resolution
D. system resolution
E. patient positioning ease
REF: 45-p. 206

1246. An adequate first pass angiocardiography study for wall motion display must be accomplished for _______ heartbeats.

A. 2-3
B. 5-6
C. 10-12
D. 20-25
E. 50-60
REF: 44-p. 273

1247. The 30° right anterior oblique position is frequently used for first pass cardiac studies as it

A. allows best momentary separation of the ventricles from the atria and aorta
B. is the most reproducible position
C. positions the face of the gamma camera closest to the patient's left ventricle
D. views the left ventricle down its long axis
E. is the easiest position for the technologist to accomplish

REF: 47-p. 129

1248. Eight to ten seconds after the administration of a radionuclide on a normal adult radionuclide angiography scan, the bolus of activity should be located entering the

A. coronary arteries
B. right atrium
C. lungs
D. left ventricle
E. descending aorta

REF: 45-p. 190

1249. Right-to-left shunts are determined visually on a radionuclide angiogram by observing

A. stasis of the radioactivity in the right ventricle
B. recirculation of the radioactivity in the lungs
C. early visualization of the left ventricle and aorta
D. nonvisualization of the right ventricle
E. collateral vessel formation around the heart

REF: 32-p. 307

1250. Quantification of the amount of right-to-left cardiac shunting may be made by determining the amount of activity distributed throughout the body after injection of

A. ^{99m}Tc sulfur colloid
B. ^{99m}Tc glucoheptonate
C. ^{99m}Tc pertechnetate
D. ^{99m}Tc macroaggregated albumin
E. ^{99m}Tc human serum albumin

REF: 44-p. 270

1251. Left-to-right shunts must have at least a __________ ratio to be detected by pulmonary/heart time activity computer generated curves.

A. 1.2:1
B. 2.0:1
C. 3.8:1
D. 4.5:1
E. 5.0:1
REF: 32-p. 309

1252. A transmission scan obtained as part of the scanning procedure for the diagnosis of pericardial effusion must be accomplished __________ the administration of a radioactive blood pool agent.

A. before
B. immediately after
C. within 1 hour
D. within 2 hours
E. after 4 hours
REF: 49-p. 87

1253. The minimum amount of fluid in a pericardial effusion necessary before radionuclide detection is

A. 10-20 ml
B. 40-50 ml
C. 100-200 ml
D. 400-500 ml
E. 1000 ml
REF: 50-p. 265

1254. The most clinically used cardiac measurement is the

A. ejection fraction
B. cardiac output
C. stroke volume
D. end-systolic volume
E. end-systolic pressure
REF: 47-p. 104

1255. The cardiac ejection fraction (EF) defined by end systolic volume (EDV) and end diastolic volume (EDV) is

A. $\frac{ESV + EDV}{ESV}$

B. $\frac{ESV + EDV}{EDV}$

C. $\frac{ESV - EDV}{ESV}$

D. $\frac{ESV - EDV}{EDV}$

E. $\frac{EDV - ESV}{EDV}$

REF: 32-p. 295

1256. The cardiac measurement defined as the blood volume pumped out by a ventricle over 1 minute is the

A. ejection fraction
B. cardiac output
C. stroke volume
D. end-systolic volume
E. end-systolic pressure
REF: 32-p. 295

1257. Stroke volume (SV) is the volume of blood ejected forward by

A. only the left ventricle during systole
B. only the right ventricle during systole
C. only the left ventricle during diastole
D. only the right ventricle during diastole
E. either ventricle during systole
F. either ventricle during diastole
REF: 47-p. 104

1258. The normal resting left ventricular ejection fraction is

A. 10-20%
B. 20-30%
C. 30-40%
D. 40-50%
E. 50-60%
REF: 48-p. 44

1259. In a graded exercise multiple gated blood pool scintigraphy a normal patient will increase his ejection fraction by about
A. 10%
B. 20%
C. 30%
D. 40%
E. 50%
REF: 43-p. 145

1260. A contraindication for performing a multiple gated equilibrium blood pool study is on a patient who
A. has atrial fibrillation (with irregular R-R intervals)
B. is pacemaker controlled
C. is unconscious
D. has less than 6 premature contractions/minute
E. is immobile
REF: 48-p. 23

1261. Paradoxical motion of a cardiac ventricular wall is described by the term
A. akinesis
B. autokinesis
C. dyskinesis
D. hyperkinesis
E. hypokinesis
REF: 44-p. 264

1262. Resting multiple gated equilibrium blood studies for assessing left ventricular wall motion are typically accomplished in the ____________ projection(s).
A. anterior
B. 45° LAO
C. 45° RAO
D. A and B
E. A and C
F. all of the above
REF: 49-p. 91

1263. Besides a gamma camera, the instrumentation required for a resting multiple gated equilibrium blood pool study is (are)
A. minicomputer
B. physiologic synchronizer (gated device)
C. 12-lead ECG device
D. A and B
E. B and C
F. all of the above
REF: 45-p. 225

1264. The most widely used signal to initiate computer data acquisition during multiple gated blood pool scintigraphy is the
A. 1st heart sound
B. 2nd heart sound
C. R wave of the electrocardiogram
D. S wave of the electrocardiogram
E. T wave of the electrocardiogram
REF: 43-p. 130

1265. The general type of collimator selected for routine multiple gated equilibrium blood pool scintigraphy is the
A. parallel hole
B. diverging
C. converging
D. single pinhole
E. multi-pinhole
REF: 43-p. 128

1266. The best radiopharmaceutical for multiple gated blood pool scintigraphy is
A. $^{99m}TcO_4^-$
B. ^{99m}Tc red blood cells (in vitro labeled)
C. ^{99m}Tc red blood cells (in vivo labeled)
D. ^{99m}Tc human serum albumin
E. ^{113m}In chloride
REF: 45-p. 227

1267. In the in vivo method of tagging red blood cells, ^{99m}Tc as pertechnetate is injected into the patient ________ after the administration of nonradioactive stannous pyrophosphate.
A. immediately
B. 10 minutes
C. 30 minutes
D. 1 hour
E. 3 hours
REF: 4-18:307, 1977

1268. The advantage of the in vivo method of labeling red blood cells over the in vitro method for gated blood pool scintigraphy is that the in vivo method
A. is more convenient to use
B. delivers less of a radiation dose
C. has a higher target-to-nontarget ratio
D. is more reliable
E. is substantially cheaper
REF: 45-p. 227

1269. In vitro ^{99m}Tc labeled red blood cells have been shown to have intravascular radioactivity retention at 30 minutes after injection of
A. 50%+
B. 60%+
C. 75%+
D. 95%+
E. 100%+
REF: 4-19:133, 1978

1270. A lead cardiac shield attached to a gamma camera's collimator before acquisition of a multiple gated equilibrium blood pool study helps the quality of the study by
A. decreasing pulse pile-up effects
B. obtaining higher target/nontarget counts
C. increasing the sensitivity of the system
D. decreasing the system dead time
E. negating object scatter effects
REF: 45-p. 225

1271. The best view for obtaining a left ventricular ejection fraction from a multiple-gated equilibrium blood-pool study is thc
A. anterior
B. 45° LAO
C. 70° LAO
D. left lateral
E. LPO
REF: 45-pp. 228-229

1272. A slight caudal tilt on a 45° LAO multiple gated equilibrium blood pool study serves to better separate the ventricles from
A. each other
B. the valve planes
C. the major vessels
D. the atria
E. the lung field
REF: 45-p. 229

1273. A clinically adequate wall motion display from a multiple gated equilibrium blood pool study requires a minimum of a ____________ computer matrix size.
A. 16 x 16
B. 32 x 32
C. 64 x 64 ← now!
D. 128 x 128
E. 256 x 256
REF: 45-p. 234

1274. On a left ventricular computer generated volume curve constructed from a LAO multiple gated equilibrium blood pool study, end-diastole occurs near the
A. first point
B. mid point
C. last point
D. A and B
E. A and C
F. all of the above
REF: 48-p. 23

1275. The typical adult dose of thallium-201 is
A. 0.5-1.0 mCi
B. 1.5-2.0 mCi
C. 3.0-4.0 mCi
D. 5.0-7.5 mCi
E. 8.5-10.0 mCi
REF: 45-p. 53

1276. In terms of blood clearance and organ distribution, thallium-201 is biologically similar to
A. cesium
B. potassium
C. gallium
D. sodium
E. magnesium
REF: 44-p. 278

1277. The myocardial kinetics of thallium after injection is described in terms of ____________ phase(s).
A. 1
B. 2
C. 3
D. 4
E. 5
REF: 45-pp. 50-51

1278. The photopeak(s) used in thallium-201 scintigraphy is (are) the
A. 69-83 keV mercury x-rays
B. 135 keV gamma ray
C. 167 keV gamma ray
D. A and B
E. A and C
F. B and C
REF: 45-p. 53

1279. Besides the anterior view, the standard views obtained in routine ^{201}Thallium scintigraphy are
A. 30° RAO and 30° and 60° LAOs
B. 30° RAO and left lateral
C. 30° RAO and LPO
D. 30° and 60° LAOs and LPO
E. left lateral and LPO
REF: 32-p. 315

1280. The optimum gamma camera imaging system for thallium-201 scintigraphy has a
A. 1/4" crystal and 19 photomultiplier tubes
B. 1/4" crystal and 37 photomultiplier tubes
C. 1/2" crystal and 19 photomultiplier tubes
D. 1/2" crystal and 37 photomultiplier tubes
E. 1/2" crystal and 61 photomultiplier tubes
REF: 45-p. 53

1281. If a cardiac collimator shield is not used during ^{201}Thallium scintigraphy, the myocardium is positioned low and to the left in the gamma camera's field of view to
A. increase the camera's count rate
B. enable the collimator to be placed as close as possible to the patient's chest
C. decrease the target-to-nontarget ratio
D. limit the number of liver counts
E. adequately image both atria
REF: 48-p. 34

1282. To avoid breast artifacts on thallium images performed on female pagients, care must be taken to
A. use only the 167 keV photopeak to reduce scatter effects
B. increase the usual dose to 3.0-4.0 mCi
C. accomplish the RAO instead of the anterior view
D. have the patient lie in the decubitus position for all views
E. tape the breast above the mediastinum
REF: 45-p. 55

1283. During thallium scintigraphy, patients lying left side up (or in the right decubitus position) for the left lateral view will
A. allow closest positioning to the detector
B. aid in the monitoring of the patient's condition
C. prevent image artifacts from photon attenuation by the diaphragm
D. permit the most reproducible position for redistribution studies
E. establish the most immobile patient position
REF: 45-p. 56

1284. The visualized portion(s) of the myocardium after ^{201}Thallium administration in a normal resting patient include
A. both atria
B. left ventricle
C. right ventricle
D. A and B
E. B and C
F. all of the above
REF: 5-7:53, 1977

1285. The central portion of a normal anterior ^{201}Thallium rest image with decreased activity represents the
A. inferior wall
B. septal wall
C. right ventricle
D. aortic arch
E. left ventricular chamber
REF: 5-7:53, 1977

1286. A focal decrease in perfusion occurring on a rest ^{201}Thallium image is most commonly caused by
A. transient myocardial ischemia
B. cardiomegaly
C. cardiogenic shock
D. previous myocardial infarction
E. cardiomyopathy
REF: 5-7:55, 1977

1287. A "cold" region found on a rest ^{201}Thallium image accomplished within 6 hours of symptoms is ________ for acute myocardial infarction.
A. sensitive and specific
B. sensitive but not specific
C. not sensitive but specific
D. not sensitive and not specific
E. either sensitive or specific
REF: 48-p. 38

1288. The sensitivity and specificity of detecting coronary artery disease (CAD) by noncomputerized planar ^{201}Thallium scintigraphy is approximately
A. 60%
B. 70%
C. 80%
D. 90%
E. 100%
REF: 45-p. 72

1289. All of the following are necessary patient preparation steps before ^{201}Thallium treadmill exercise scintigraphy begins EXCEPT
A. placement of standard ECG monitor leads
B. NPO orders for at least 6 hours before testing
C. stopping digitalis preparations 2 days previous to testing
D. placement of an intravenous infusion of 5% dextrose in water in a hand or forearm vein
E. a thorough explanation of the treadmill and thallium imaging procedure
REF: 48-p. 31

1290. If at all possible, a patient should continue to exercise for at least ____________ following dose administration in ^{201}Thallium scintigraphy.
A. 30 seconds
B. 90 seconds
C. 2 minutes
D. 3 minutes
E. No further exercise is required
REF: 5-7:50, 1977

1291. In order to consistently detect regions of reversibly ischemic, myocardial regions ^{201}Thallium imaging must begin within ____________ minutes after the treadmill stress study and be completed within __________ minutes.
A. 5; 10
B. 5; 30
C. 20; 30
D. 20; 45
E. 30; 45
REF: 48-p. 34

1292. Approximately ____________% of administered thallium-201 localizes in the myocardium immediately after a stress study.

A. 4
B. 10
C. 16
D. 22
E. 28
REF: 45-p. 52

1293. On a normal stress thallium-201 study, over 50% of patients have decreased activity to the ____________ region of the myocardium on the anterior image.

A. septal
B. lateral
C. inferior
D. superior
E. apical
REF: 5-7:54, 1977

1294. Transient myocardial ischemia appears as a focal ____________ lesion on initial stress ^{201}Thallium images which ____________ on 4-hour delay images.

A. "cold"; remains "cold"
B. "cold"; becomes "hot"
C. "cold"; becomes normal
D. "hot"; remains "hot"
E. "hot"; becomes "cold"
F. "hot"; becomes normal
REF: 48-p. 31

1295. The digital minicomputer used as part of thallium scintigraphy provides

A. image enhancement
B. quantification analysis
C. automatic diagnosis
D. A and B
E. B and C
F. all of the above
REF: 44-p. 421

1296. The use of the seven pinhole collimator or the slant hole collimator attached to high resolution gamma camera systems for performing ^{201}Thallium scintigraphy has introduced

A. improved system sensitivity
B. improved system linearity
C. improved system resolution
D. easier positioning techniques
E. tomographic myocardium images
REF: 45-p. 58

1297. The major disadvantage of imaging the myocardium with intracoronary injection of ^{99m}Technetium labeled particles is the

A. high background that is difficult to eliminate
B. invasiveness of the procedure
C. tendency of the particles to break down in arterial blood
D. high possibility of a technically inadequate study
E. high dose of radiopharmaceutical required
REF: 45-p. 108

1298. Intracoronary injection of ^{133}Xenon performed during diagnostic coronary arteriography is primarily used to obtain quantitative information about

A. pulmonary artery flow
B. coronary artery stenosis
C. regional capillary blood flow
D. myocardium mass
E. extent of myocardial infarction
REF: 45-p. 119

1299. Peripheral arterial vascular disease may be evaluated by scintigraphic methods using the following radiopharmaceuticals

A. ^{99m}Tc MAA
B. ^{99m}Tc DTPA
C. ^{133}Xe
D. A and B
E. A and C
F. all of the above
REF: 43-p. 350

1300. ^{99m}Tc MAA or ^{99m}Tc HAM used in the study of peripheral circulation are used for the determination of

A. arterial perfusion
B. blood pool volume
C. blood flow per gram of tissue
D. blood clearance
E. tissue diffusion
REF: 50-p. 302

1301. The administration technique used with ^{133}Xe for the nonimaging probe evaluation of peripheral vascular disease is

A. inhalation of a small volume of ^{133}Xe as a gas
B. peripheral intravenous injection of ^{133}Xe dissolved in saline
C. peripheral intravenous injection of a small volume of ^{133}Xe as a gas
D. oral administration of ^{133}Xe dissolved in saline
E. intramuscular injectionof ^{133}Xe dissolved in saline
REF: 43-p. 353

1302. The most recent radiolabel used in the fibrinogen uptake test used for thrombophlebitis detection is

A. ^{123}I
B. ^{124}I
C. ^{125}I
D. ^{127}I
E. ^{131}I
REF: 32-p. 318

1303. The limitation(s) of the ^{125}I fibrinogen uptake test related to the low energy photon is (are)

A. state-of-the-art computerization is required to adequately image distribution of fibrinogen
B. pelvic or upper thigh are excluded from examination
C. imaging techniques cannot be done to demonstrate uptake of the fibrinogen
D. A and B
E. A and C
F. B and C
REF: 45-p. 348

1304. The ____________ labeled fibrinogen test allows discrimination of deposition of fibrinogen within vascular channels from areas of cellulitis, hematomas, and arthritis.

A. ^{123}I
B. ^{124}I
C. ^{125}I
D. ^{131}I
E. ^{99m}Tc
REF: 45-p. 349

1305. An area of the leg is considered abnormal determined by the ^{125}I fibrinogen uptake study when the counts are at least ____________% higher than adjacent areas on the same leg.

A. 20%
B. 35%
C. 50%
D. 65%
E. 80%
REF: 32-p. 321

1306. For radionuclide venography, all of the following rules should be followed EXCEPT

A. gently invert the ^{99m}Tc MAA several times before injection
B. avoid a bubble introduction while administering the dose
C. avoid drawing back blood in the radionuclide syringes
D. use 3–5 ml of normal saline as a flush behind the ^{99m}Tc MAA
E. periodically flush the administration system with heparin to keep the system free
REF: 32-p. 323

1307. The usual dose of ^{99m}Tc MAA or ^{99m}Tc HAM in each syringe for radionuclide venography is

A. 0.5–1.0 mCi
B. 2.0–3.0 mCi
C. 5.0–7.0 mCi
D. 8.0–10.0 mCi
E. 15.0–20.0 mCi
REF: 36-p. 473

1308. Before ^{99m}Tc MAA is administered in radionuclide venography, tourniquets are applied above the
A. ankles
B. knees
C. thighs
D. A and B
E. A and C
F. B and C
REF: 36-p. 473

1309. The presence of collateral flow around deep venous circulation on a ^{99m}Tc MAA venography exam most likely indicates
A. cellulitis
B. hemangioma
C. hematoma
D. occlusion
E. arthritis
REF: 45-p. 374

1310. Visualization of both the superficial saphenous and deep venous system during radionuclide venography is indicative of
A. too large a volume of injected radiopharmaceutical
B. a positive study for thrombophlebitis
C. not enough pressure exerted when administering the dose
D. bifurcation of the saphenous vein
E. the ankle tourniquet not being applied tight enough
REF: 45-p. 369

20. MISCELLANEOUS PROCEDURES

DIRECTIONS: Each of the questions or incomplete statements below is followed by a list of suggested answers or completions. Select the **one** that is **BEST** in each case.

1311. Carrier-free ^{67}Gallium has an effective half-life of about ____________ hours and a physical half-life of ____________ days.

A. 40; 3.25
B. 40; 5.3
C. 70; 3.25
D. 70; 5.3
E. 100; 3.25
F. 100; 5.3
REF: 32-p. 423

1312. What organ accumulates the greatest percent of injected ^{67}Ga citrate dose per gram of tissue as determined by autopsy studies?

A. Spleen
B. Lymph nodes
C. Stomach
D. Heart
E. Brain
REF: 4-13(1):92, 1972

1313. ^{67}Ga citrate normally localizes in the patient's liver, spleen, and
A. bone
B. myocardium
C. colon
D. A and B
E. A and C
F. B and C
REF: 14-p. 157

1314. At 24 hours approximately ____________% of injected ^{67}Ga citrate is excreted in the urine of a normal patient.
A. 2-5
B. 10-15
C. 20-25
D. 30-35
E. 40-45
REF: 32-p. 423

1315. The increased presence of ^{67}Ga in the ____________ at 48 hours post dose administration is considered an abnormal finding.
A. kidneys
B. liver
C. spleen
D. colon
E. bone marrow
REF: 8:230, 1978

1316. A scintillation camera equipped with a parallel hole collimator rated to at least ____________ keV should be used for selected ^{67}Gallium citrate images.
A. 100
B. 150
C. 200
D. 300
E. 400
REF: 32-p. 429

1317. What energy peaks of ^{67}Ga should be used on a dual PHA gamma camera for detection of a suspected abdominal deep lesion in an obese patient?
A. 93 keV, 184 keV
B. 93 keV, 296 keV
C. 93 keV, 388 keV
D. 184 keV, 296 keV
E. 296 keV, 388 keV
REF: 14-p. 158

1318. The main difference in ^{67}Ga citrate distribution between normal adult and normal pediatric patients is that the latter have increased radiopharmaceutical concentration in the
A. transverse colon
B. epiphyseal plates of growing bones
C. kidneys, ureters, and bladder
D. soft tissue of the extremities
E. metabolic active areas of the liver
REF: 4-18(11):1057, 1977

1319. All of the following are advantages of ^{67}Ga scintigraphy over ultrasonography in abscess detection EXCEPT ^{67}Ga scintigraphy is
A. a survey exam which can include all portions of the body
B. less dependent on operator expertise
C. more easily accomplished on patients with drainage wounds or with overlying bandages
D. quickly accomplished after radionuclide injection
E. highly sensitive for formed (abscess) and less well confined (peritonitis) lesions
REF: 14-p. 164

1320. The overall sensitivity and specificity of ^{67}Ga citrate in the detection of abdominal inflammatory disease is about
A. 50%
B. 60%
C. 70%
D. 80%
E. 90%
REF: 14-p. 163

1321. The proper patient positioning for ^{67}Ga abscess scintigraphy performed on a large field of view camera with whole-body-imaging capability is
A. prone, from midchest to midpelvis
B. prone, from top of the head to midpelvis
C. supine, from top of the head to midchest
D. supine, from midchest to midthigh
E. supine, from top of the head to midthigh
REF: 32-p. 428

1322. Patients injected with ^{67}Ga may be effectively scanned as early as 6 hours after dose administration as an aid in the diagnosis of
A. pulmonary metastases
B. abdominal abscess
C. Hodgkin's disease
D. viral pneumonia
E. liver carcinoma
REF: 4-16(11):990, 1975

1323. Large ____________ usually appear on ^{67}Ga images as distinct focal "cold" areas.
A. hematomas
B. hepatomas
C. myocardial infarcts
D. region of osteomyelitis
E. pneumonias
REF: 5-8:230, 1978

1324. Which of the following benign disease processes avidly concentrates ^{67}Ga citrate and is therefore evaluated by its use?
A. Hemangioma
B. Lipoma
C. Sarcoidosis
D. Pancreatitis
E. Thyroiditis
REF: 36-p. 548

1325. The left adrenal gland lies more ____________ and ____________ than the right adrenal gland.
A. anterior; lateral
B. anterior; inferior
C. anterior; superior
D. posterior; lateral
E. posterior; inferior
F. posterior; superior
REF: 32-p. 258

1326. Routine protocols for ^{131}I iodocholesterol adrenal scintigraphy should include serial imaging with camera/ computer images of 50,000 counts or acquired for a period of
A. 30 seconds
B. 5 minutes
C. 20 minutes
D. 40 minutes
E. 1 hour
REF: 36-p. 572

1327. Technical reasons which can be responsible for the absence of ^{131}I radiocholesterol in the adrenal glands of normal patients include all of the following EXCEPT
A. the use of medium energy collimation instead of a low energy all purpose collimator
B. breakdown of the radiolabel due to excessive exposure to heat and light
C. previous corticosteroid medication
D. incorrect patient positioning
E. extravasation of the radiopharmaceutical
REF: 5-8:23, 1978

1328. The technical quality of ^{131}I iodocholesterol adrenal scintigraphy accomplished on a patient with suspected primary aldosteronism may be improved by
A. performing an adrenal uptake of the iodocholesterol
B. pretreating the patient with Lugol's solution
C. dexamethasone suppression of ACTH before imaging begins
D. A and B
E. A and C
F. all of the above
REF: 5-8:23, 1978

1329. Hyperparathyroidism is best evaluated by a nuclear medicine double tracer technique using the radiopharmaceuticals

A. ^{131}I and $^{99m}TcO_4^-$
B. $^{99m}TcO_4^-$ and ^{201}Tl
C. ^{201}Tl and ^{131}Cs
D. ^{131}Cs and $^{99m}TcO_4^-$
E. ^{131}Cs and ^{131}I
REF: 4-24:438, 1983

1330. Double tracer parathyroid scintigraphy is most successfully accomplished using a gamma camera equipped with a

A. pinhold collimator and an on-line minicomputer
B. pinhold collimator and a physiologic gating device
C. general purpose parallel hole collimator and a video tape recorder
D. high resolution parallel hole collimator and a physiologic gating device
E. high resolution parallel hole collimator and a video tape recorder
REF: 4-24:438, 1983

1331. The radiopharmaceutical of choice for testicular scintigraphy is

A. ^{67}Ga citrate
B. ^{99m}Tc sulfur colloid
C. ^{99m}Tc as pertechnetate
D. ^{99m}Tc DTPA
E. ^{111}In WBCs
REF: 32-p. 359

1332. The patient is asked to empty his bladder before $^{99m}TcO_4^-$ testicular scintigraphy begins to

A. reduce the radiation dose to the bladder and surrounding tissue
B. enhance the perfusion to the testes, which may be decreased due to a full bladder
C. avoid localization of the $^{99m}TcO_4^-$ which could interfere with visual interpretation
D. prevent discomfort during this long procedure
E. shorten the required time for $^{99m}TcO_4^-$ rium within the vascular compartment
REF: 53-p. 243

1333. Acute epididymitis characteristically appears on $^{99m}TcO_4^-$ testicular scrintigraphy as
A. a normal flow study but increased testicular activity on the static images
B. a decreased flow study but a normal static study
C. a decreased flow study but with increased testicular activity on the static images
D. an increased flow study with increased testicular activity on the static images
E. an increased flow study but with decreased activity on the static images
REF: 58-p. 374

1334. A finding of decreased perfusion on dynamic images and decreased testicular activity on the static images of a $^{99m}TcO_4^-$ testicular study is indicative of
A. a normal scan
B. chronic epididymitis
C. tumor
D. acute torsion
E. a spermatocele
REF: 53-p. 239

1335. In testicular scintigraphy, which of the following would cause increased $^{99m}TcO_4^-$ uptake in the testes on both dynamic and static blood pool images?
A. Epididymitis
B. Torsion
C. Vascular tumors
D. A and B
E. A and C
F. All of the above
REF: 53-p. 237

1336. ^{111}In labeled white blood cells (WBCs) offers all of the following advantages for the detection of abdominal abscess EXCEPT it
A. has a half-life which allows sequential scanning over several days
B. is technically easy to perform imaging with the use of a whole body table equipped gamma camera
C. can be performed quickly after ^{111}In WBCs administration to the patient
D. has a high target-to-nontarget ratio for abscess
E. can be useful in the detection of extraabdominal sources of sepsis
REF: 8-140:155, 1981

1337. Which of the following steps are required for ^{111}In labeling of leukocytes?
A. Separation of the leukocytes from the platelets and red blood cells
B. Incubation of the leukocytes with ^{111}In oxine
C. Separation of labeled cells from any other radioactivity
D. A and B
E. B and C
F. All of the above
REF: 4-21:122, 1980

1338. The normal distribution of ^{111}In labeled leukocytes in man at 24 hours after administration is primarily within
A. muscle, lungs, and bone marrow
B. muscle, liver, and lungs
C. liver, spleen, and bone marrow
D. liver, spleen, and lungs
E. spleen, muscle, and bone marrow
REF: 4-18:1014, 1977

1339. ^{111}In labeled white blood cells may first become apparent in inflammatory sites ____________ after patient administration of the radioactive cells.
A. immediately
B. 15 minutes
C. 60 minutes
D. 4 hours
E. 24 hours
REF: 4-18:1014, 1977

1340. Possible pitfalls which can mimic foci of sepsis in ^{111}In leukocyte scintigraphy include all of the following EXCEPT
A. accessory spleens
B. overlying bowel activity
C. clumping of the leukocytes previous to administration
D. previous radiation therapy
E. myocardial or cerebral infarction
REF: 4-21:122, 1980

1341. The organ receiving the largest radiation dose from ^{111}In labeled platelets is the
A. spleen
B. liver
C. lung
D. kidneys
E. gonads
REF: 8-140:169, 1981

1342. Lymphoscintigraphy is a useful diagnostic tool for all of the following indications EXCEPT
A. staging of known Hodgkin's disease
B. study of lymphatic leukemia
C. evaluation of lymphatic kinetics
D. anatomical sizing of lymph nodes
E. search for metastatic invasion of the lymph nodes

1343. The radiopharmaceutical of choice for lymphoscintigraphy is
A. ^{99m}Tc antimony sulfide
B. ^{99m}Tc Sn phytate
C. ^{99m}Tc sulfur colloid
D. ^{198}Au colloid
E. ^{99m}Tc DTPA
REF: 4-20:933, 1979

1344. Lymphoscintigraphy of the abdominal lymph nodes begins with an injection of radiocolloid

A. intravenously in a superficial vein of the foot
B. intramuscularly in the calf muscles of both legs
C. subcutaneously in the interdigital webs of the feet
D. intravenously in both femoral veins
E. intraperitonealy on both lateral sides of the abdomen

REF: 50-p. 327

1345. The results of injecting relatively large particles (> 100 microns) of ^{99m}Tc tagged particles for lymphoscintigraphy are

A. rapid absorption within the liver
B. "hangup" of the activity at the injection site
C. quicker breakdown of the "tag" from the colloid
D. possible allergic reaction to the patient
E. transport through the lymph chain speeded too quickly for camera acquisition

REF: 36-p. 579

1346. Possible pitfalls in the interpretation of parasternal lymphoscintigraphy include all of the following EXCEPT

A. the possibility of contralateral migration of the radiopharmaceutical
B. the fact that anatomical symmetry is not always present
C. the existence of a solitary lymphatic chain behind or on either side of the sternum
D. uptake of activity in normal comparable nodes may differ
E. the relatively small proportion of the activity localizing in the liver instead of transported by the lymphatics

REF: 50-p. 326

1347. Positive ^{99m}Tc RBCs scintigraphy for the detection of liver hemangioma characteristically appears as a(n) __________ dynamic study with __________ focal localization on the 6-hour static study.
A. normal; decreased
B. normal; increased
C. increased; decreased
D. increased; increased
E. decreased; decreased
REF: 3-12:119, 1984

1348. The radiopharmaceutical of choice for determination of LeVeen shunt patency is
A. ^{99m}Tc DTPA
B. ^{99m}Tc PYP
C. ^{99m}Tc Sulfur colloid
D. ^{99m}Tc RBCs
E. ^{99m}Tc GHA
REF: 36-p. 575

1349. The route of radiopharmaceutical administration for evaluation of LeVeen shunt patency is
A. intravenous
B. intraperitoneal
C. intramuscular
D. subcutaneous
E. oral
REF: 36-p. 575

1350. A functioning LeVeen shunt determined by nuclear scintigraphy is indicated when
A. the shunt tubing is visualized in the anterior thoracic wall
B. the liver and the spleen are visualized in the abdomen
C. diffuse activity accumulates below the diaphragm
D. A and B
E. B and C
F. all of the above
REF: 4-18:29, 1977

1351. The ^{32}P procedure used for screening malignancies of the eye requires the use of a
A. specialized G-M probe
B. sensitive "cutie pie"
C. pinhole equipped gamma camera
D. dual head rectilinear scanner
E. deep well counter
REF: 36-p. 552

1352. The images acquired during $^{99m}TcO_4^-$ dacryocystography are accomplished on a gamma camera equipped with a ____________ collimator.
A. pinhole
B. converging
C. diverging
D. focused
E. general purpose
REF: 58-p. 309

1353. The patient positioning for nuclear dacryosystography using $^{99m}TcO_4^-$ is
A. upright
B. supine
C. prone
D. A or B
E. B or C
F. A or B or C
REF: 58-p. 309

1354. Normally functioning lacrimal drainage apparatus is indicated by nuclear dacryocystography when
A. both eyes concentrate activity
B. activity is located in the nose area within 15 minutes
C. activity is located in nose area at 4-6 hours
D. the thyroid localizes activity within 15 minutes
E. the thyroid localizes activity at 4-6 hours
REF: 36-p. 562

1355. I-131 therapy for thyroid disease is used to treat
A. hyperthyroidism
B. hypothyroidism
C. thyroid carcinoma
D. A and B
E. A and C
F. all of the above
REF: 65-p. 711

1356. The greatest variable in the estimation of a physiologically appropriate therapeutic dose of ^{131}I is
A. the percent uptake
B. the biologic half-life
C. the effective half-life
D. the weight and shape of the gland
E. the number of cold nodules in the gland
REF: 65-p. 718

1357. A single-dose treatment of hyperthyroidism with ^{131}I requires approximately
A. 100 μCi
B. 8 mCi
C. 20 mCi
D. 50 mCi
E. 100 mCi
REF: 65-p. 715

1358. A contraindication for ^{131}I therapy for thyroid disease is
A. pregnancy
B. recent myocardial infarction
C. diabetes
D. A and B
E. A and C
F. all of the above
REF: 65-p. 712

1359. The most common complication of ^{131}I therapy is
A. cardiac failure
B. ocular disorder
C. myxedema
D. induction of leukemia
E. hypertension
REF: 65-p. 715

1360. Although many dose schedules have been devised for ^{131}I treatment of metastatic thyroid carcinoma, the largest dose usually administered is
A. 50 mCi
B. 100 mCi
C. 150 mCi
D. 200 mCi
E. 250 mCi
REF: 65-p. 738

1361. The limiting factor for ^{131}I treatment of metastatic thyroid carcinoma is usually
A. bone marrow effects
B. genetic damage
C. liver damage
D. salivary gland damage
E. leukemia inducement
REF: 65-p. 740

1362. Polycythemia vera is a ____________ syndrome.
A. benign
B. neoplastic
C. acquired
D. extremely rare
E. pediatric
REF: 65-p. 761

1363. An early manifestation of polycythemia vera is
A. a decrease in liver function
B. an increase in thyroid size
C. an increase in red cell production
D. loss of functioning marrow from the bone
E. metastatic invasion of bone marrow
REF: 65-p. 761

1364. The initial dose of ^{32}P used to treat polycythemia vera is usually
A. 300 μCi
B. 3 mCi
C. 30 mCi
D. 300 mCi
E. 330 mCi
REF: 65-p. 765

1365. P-32 given for treatment of polycythemia vera is normally given by
A. mouth
B. parenteral injection
C. intravenous injection
D. intramuscular injection
E. subcutaneous injection
REF: 65-p. 761

1366. Intracavitary therapy with radiocolloids is used to treat
A. uterine cancer
B. brain tumors
C. malignant effusions
D. prostate cancer
E. leukemia
REF: 65-p. 777

REFERENCES

1. Early, P. J., Razzak, M. A., Sodee, D. B.: *Textbook of Nuclear Medicine Technology,* 3rd Edition. C. V. Mosby Co., St. Louis, 1979

2. Medical Internal Radiation Dose Committee (MIRD) Pamphlets, Published as JNM: *Journal of Nuclear Medicine Supplements*

3. *Journal of Nuclear Medicine Technology,* published by the Society of Nuclear Medicine, New York

4. *Journal of Nuclear Medicine,* published by the Society of Nuclear Medicine, New York

5. *Seminars in Nuclear Medicine,* published by Grune & Stratton, Inc., New York

6. National Council on Radiation Protection and Measurements, NCRP #37: *Precautions in the Management of Patients Who Have Received Therapeutic Amounts of Radionuclides,* Washington, D. C., 1970

7. National Council on Radiation Protection and Measurements, NCRP #39: *Basic Radiation Protection Criteria,* Washington, D. C., 1971

8. *Radiology,* published by the Radiological Society of North America, Easton, PA

9. Rhodes, B. C. (Ed.): *Quality Control in Nuclear Medicine.* C. V. Mosby Co., St. Louis, 1977

10. Rollo, F. D. (Ed.): *Nuclear Medicine Physics Instrumentation and Agents.* C. V. Mosby Co., St. Louis, 1977

11. Coulam, C. M., Erickson, J. J., Rollo, F. D., James, A. E. Jr.: *Medical Imaging.* Appleton-Century-Crofts, New York, 1981

12. Sorenson, J. A. and Phelps, M. E.: *Physics in Nuclear Medicine.* Grune & Stratton, New York, 1980

13. Hoffer, P. B., Beckerman, C., Henkin, R. E.: *Gallium-67 Imaging.* John Wiley & Sons, New York, 1978

14. Alavi, A. and Arger, P. (Eds.): *Multiple Imaging Procedures,* Vol. 3. Grune & Stratton, New York, 1980

15. Rothfeld, B.: *Nuclear Medicine: Hepatolienal.* J. B. Lippincott Co., Philadelphia, 1980

16. Pick, T. P. and Howden, R. (Eds.): *Gray's Anatomy.* Bounty Books, New York, 1977

17. Matin, P.: *Handbook of Clinical Nuclear Medicine.* Medical Examination Publishing Co., Inc., Garden City, New York, 1981

18. Wagner, H. N. Jr. (Ed.): *Nuclear Medicine.* H. P. Publishing Co., New York, 1975

19. Bushong, S. C.: *Radiologic Science for Technologists; Physics, Biology & Protection,* 2nd Ed. C. V. Mosby Co., St. Louis, 1983

20. Marriott, H. J. L.: *Practical Electrocardiography,* 6th Edition. Williams & Wilkins Co., Baltimore, Md., 1977

21. Blowers, M. G. and Smith, R. J. (Eds.): *How To Read An ECG Basic Interpretation for Nurses and Other Health Workers,* Revised Edition. Medical Economics Co., New Jersey, 1980

22. Horrobin, D. F.: *An Introduction to Human Physiology.* F. A. Davis Co., Philadelphia, 1973

23. Dalrymple, G. B., Gaulden, M. E., Kollmorgen, G. M., Vogel, H. H. (Eds.): *Medical Radiation Biology.* W. B. Saunders Co., Philadelphia, 1973

24. Pizzarells, D. J. and Witcofski, R. L.: *Medical Radiation Biology,* Third Edition. Lea & Febiger, Philadelphia, 1982

25. Casarett, A. P.: *Radiation Biology.* Prentice-Hall, Inc., Englewood Cliffs, N. J., 1968

26. Behrens, C. F., King, E. R., Carpender, J. W. J.: *Atomic Medicine,* 5th Edition. Williams & Wilkins Co., Baltimore, 1969

27. Travis, E. L.: *Primer of Medical Radiobiology.* Year Book Medical Publishers, Chicago, 1975

28. Coggle, J. E.: *Biological Effects of Radiation.* Wykeham Publication, London, 1971

29. Ducan, W. and Nias, A. H. W.: *Clinical Radiobiology.* Churchill Livingstone, Edinburgh, 1977

30. Hall, E. J.: *Radiobiology for the Radiologist,* 2nd Edition. Harper & Row, Hagerstown, 1978

31. Spencer, R. P.: *Nuclear Medicine: Focus on Clinical Diagnosis,* 2nd Edition. Medical Examination Publishing Co., Inc., 1977

32. Bernier, D., Langan, J., Wells, L. D. (Eds.): *Nuclear Medicine Technology and Techniques.* C. V. Mosby Co., St. Louis, 1981

33. Schneider, P. B. and Treves, S. (Eds.): *Nuclear Medicine in Clinical Practice.* Elsevier/North-Holland Biomedical Press, New York, 1978

34. Odell, W. D. and Franchimont, P.: *Principles of Competitive Protein-Binding Assays,* 2nd Edition. John Wiley & Sons, New York, 1983

35. Ashkar, F., Miale, A., Smoak, W.: *A Study Guide in Nuclear Medicine.* Charles C. Thomas, Publishers, Springfield, Illinois, 1975

36. Sodee, D. B. and Early, P. J.: *Mosby's Manual of Nuclear Medicine Procedures,* 3rd Edition. C. V. Mosby Co., St. Louis, 1981

37. Andrews, J. T. and Milne, M. J.: *Nuclear Medicine: Clinical and Technological Basis.* John Wiley & Sons, New York, 1977

38. Greenfield, L. D. and Uszler, J. M.: *Nuclear Medicine in Clinical Practice: Selective Correlations with Ultrasound and CT,* Verlag Chemic International, Inc., Deerfield Beach, Florida, 1982

39. *Physician's Desk Reference for Radiology and Nuclear Medicine.* Charles E. Baker, J. Litton Industries, Inc., 1979/80

40. Rothfeld, B. (Ed.): *Nuclear Medicine In Vitro,* 2nd Edition. J. B. Lippincott Company, New York, 1983

41. Werner, S. C. and Ingbar, S. H. (Eds.): *The Thyroid: A Fundamental and Clinical Text,* 4th Edition. Harper and Row, New York, 1978

42. Keyes, J. W. Jr. (Ed.): *CRC Manual of Nuclear Medicine Procedures,* 3rd Edition. CRC Press, West Palm Beach, Florida, 1978

43. Strauss, H. W. and Pitt, B. (Eds.): *Cardiovascular Nuclear Medicine,* 2nd Edition. C. V. Mosby Co., St. Louis, Mo, 1979

44. Holman, B. L. and Parker, J. A. (Eds.): *Computer-Assisted Cardiac Nuclear Medicine,* First Edition. Little, Brown and Co., Inc., Boston, 1981

45. Berman, D. S. and Mason, D. T. (Eds.): *Clinical Nuclear Cardiology.* Grune & Stratton, Inc., New York, 1981

46. Grossman, Z. D., Ellis, D. A., Brigham, S. C. (Eds.): *The Clinician's Guide to Diagnostic Imaging.* Raven Press, New York, 1983

47. Mettler, F. A. and Guiberteau, M. J. (Eds.): *Essentials Of Nuclear Medicine Imaging.* Grune & Stratton, New York, 1983

48. Sprengelmeyer, J. and Weisberger, C. L.: *Practical Nuclear Cardiology.* Harper & Row, 1979

49. Clifton, N. A. and Simmons, P. J. (Eds.): *Basic Imaging Procedures in Nuclear Medicine.* Appleton-Century-Crofts, New York, 1981

50. Rocha, A. F. G. and Harbert, J. C. (Eds.): *Textbook of Nuclear Medicine: Clinical Applications.* Lea & Febiger, Philadelphia, 1979

51. Baum, S. and Bramlet, R. (Eds.): *Basic Nuclear Medicine.* Appleton-Century-Crofts, New York, 1975

52. Ell, P. J. and Williams, E. S. (Eds.): *Nuclear Medicine: An Introductory Text,* 1st Ed. Blackwell Scientific Publications, Oxford, 1981

53. Walker, J. M. and Margouleff, D. (Eds.): *A Clinical Manual of Nuclear Medicine.* Appleton-Century-Crofts, Norwalk, Conn., 1984

54. *Clinical Nuclear Medicine.* J. B. Lippincott Co., Philadelphia

55. Rhodes, B. A. and Croft, B. Y. (Eds.): *Basics of Radiopharmacy.* C. V. Mosby Co., St. Louis, 1978

56. Maisey, M. N., Britton, K. E., Gilday, D. L. (Eds.): *Clinical Nuclear Medicine.* W. B. Saunders Co., Philadelphia, 1983

57. Handmaker, H. and Lowenstein, J. M. (Eds.): *Nuclear Medicine in Clinical Pediatrics.* The Society of Nuclear Medicine, New York, 1975

58. Kirchner, P. T.: *Nuclear Medicine Review Syllabus.* The Society of Nuclear Medicine, New York, 1980

59. Sodee, D. B. and Early, P. J.: *Technology and the Interpretation of Nuclear Medicine Procedures,* 3rd Edition. C. V. Mosby Co., St. Louis, 1979

60. *American Journal Roentgenology, Radium Therapy, and Nuclear Medicine,* published by Charles C. Thomas, Springfield, Ill.

61. *Vignettes in Nuclear Medicine,* Brucer, M., published by Mallinckrodt Chemical Works, St. Louis

62. Kereiakes, J. G. and Corey, K. R.: *AAPM Monograph No. 1. Biophysical Aspects of the Medical Use of Technetium-99m,* AAPM Committee on Nuclear Medicine, 1976

63. Sarper, R. M.: *Nuclear Medicine Instrumentation.* Charles C. Thomas, Springfield, Ill, 1984

64. Blahd, W. H.: *Nuclear Medicine,* 2nd Edition. McGraw-Hill Book Co., New York, 1971

ANSWERS AND COMMENTS

The authors and the publisher of this book have made every effort to thoroughly verify the answers to the questions which appear on the preceding pages. However, as in any text, some inaccuracies and ambiguities may occur; therefore, if in doubt, please consult your references.

The Publisher

1. C. Radioactive means that the material emits radiation.

2. C. Light, x-rays, and neutrinos are all massless.

3. C. Atoms combine in a specific way to form a molecule. For example, two hydrogen atoms and one oxygen atom form a water molecule (H_2O).

4. B. If you divide a molecule into its constituent atoms, its physical properties change.

5. D. All the atoms of a single type are called an element.

6. B. Periodic table - groups of families of elements.

7. C. The e.V. is a unit of energy.

8. B. Potential energy is the energy of position.

9. B. An angstrom is 10^{-8} cm.

10. B. Coulomb first put the law in its mathematical form.

11. B. Unlike charges attract each other.

12. B. Photon is the word for a single unit (or quantum) of electromagnetic energy.

13. A. Electromagnetic radiation can always be thought of as a wave.

14. C. This is the definition of wavelength.

15. C. Frequency *times* wavelength is equal to the speed of light.

16. A. Longer since its energy is less.

17. B. Lower since its energy is less.

18. B. Since $\lambda = c/\nu$, if ν is larger, c/ν becomes smaller.

19. A. This is the definition of the velocity of a wave.

20. B. This is the definition of frequency.

21. A. All electromagnetic radiation travels with this velocity in free space. However, the velocity is less in matter.

22. A. Energy is proportional to frequency.

23. B. Planck discovered some of the fundamental properties of radiation.

24. D. $E = h\nu$; $\lambda\nu = c$; $\nu = c/\lambda$ $E = hc/\lambda$

25. A. 12,400 is hc in eV-Angstroms.

26. D. $E = h\nu$; $E = 4.13 \times 10^{-18}$ 5.6×10^{19}; $E = 231$ keV.

27. C. $E = hc/\lambda$; $E = 12.4 \times 10^{-8}/21 \times 10^{-9}$; $E = 59$ keV.

28. D. $E = hc/\lambda$; $E = 12.4 \times 10^{-8}/13 \times 10^{-9}$ $E = 9.5$ keV.

29. A. $E = hc/\lambda$; $\lambda = hc/E$; $\lambda = 12.4 \times 10^{-8}/175$; $\lambda = 7 \times 10^{-10}$ cm.

30. C. $\nu = c/\lambda$; $\nu = 3 \times 10^{10}/5.7 \times 10^{-12}$; $\nu = 5.3 \times 10^{21}$ Hz.

31. D. $\nu = c/\lambda$; $\nu = 3.0 \times 10^{10}/5 \times 10^{-5}$; $\nu = 6 \times 10^{14}$ Hz.

32. C. $\lambda = c/\nu$; $\nu = 3 \times 10^{10}/2.5 \times 10^{20}$; $\nu = 1.2 \times 10^{-10}$ cm.

33. B. $E = \frac{hc}{\lambda}$; $\lambda = \frac{hc}{E} = \frac{12.4 \times 10^{-8}}{8} = 15.4 \times 10^{-9}$

34. A. $E = h\nu$; $\nu = E/h$; $\nu = 35/4.13 \times 10^{-18}$; $\nu = 8.5 \times 10^{18}$ Hz.

35. B. $E = h\nu$; $E = 4.13 \times 10^{-18}\ 1.36 \times 10^{20}$; $E = 562$ keV.

36. B. $E = h\nu$; $\nu = E/h$; $\nu = 100/4.13 \times 10^{-18}$; $\nu = 24 \times 10^{18}$ Hz.

37. B. $\nu = c/\lambda$; $\nu = 3 \times 10^{10}/12 \times 10^{18}$; $\nu = 2.5 \times 10^{-9}$ cm.

38. A. The different manifestations of electromagnetic radiation are due to differences in energy, frequency, and wavelength.

39. B. X-rays are associated with electrons; γ-rays with the nucleus. All the other properties (e.g., charge, mass, velocity) are the same.

40. D. An α-particle is a $^{4}_{2}He$ nucleus. They have mass. Gamma rays have no mass.

41. D. The only difference between gamma rays and x-rays is their origin.

42. B. Gamma rays carry no charge.

43. B. An ion is an electrically charged particle.

44. A. The electron is given more energy but it is not removed from the atom.

45. C. The removal of electrons from atoms is called ionization.

46. D. Both are true, since it takes different amounts of energy to remove electrons from different shells and each shell represents an energy level.

47. D. $2N^2$ rule; $2 \times 2^2 = 8$

48. B. The shells are K, L, M. The K is closest to the nucleus.

49. A. K-shell holds 2 electrons, helium has 2 electrons.

50. A. Filled in most stable; + or - one electron is most reactive.

51. D. For example, L = 2; $2(2)^2 = 8$

52. C. This is because M-shell binding energies are less than L-shell binding energies.

53. C. Energy = binding energy final minus binding energy initial. So 70 - 8 = 62 keV.

54. B. Exactly 33 keV.

55. B. This is the famous law for changing matter into energy.

56. B. Individual nuclei decay in a random fashion. The probability of decay is controlled by the decay constant.

57. D. The binding energy for nuclei is reflected as a loss of mass.

58. C. The binding energy shows up as a loss of mass from $E = mc^2$.

59. C. Since ^{32}P and ^{32}S both have the same number of nucleons.

60. C. The mass is lost as binding energy.

61. B. Isotopes have same proton number (Z), same chemical properties; but different mass number (A).

62. D. The atomic weight (or mass) is what distinguishes isotopes.

63. C. Most of the mass of an atom is in the nucleus.

64. D. Stable nuclei usually have more neutrons than protons.

65. D. The rate of radioactive decay cannot be altered by any common physical or chemical means.

66. C. This is the definition of an excited state.

67. C. Gamma emission and internal conversion are the two competing processes.

68. B. Gamma emission doesn't change the mass number (A) or the charge (Z).

69. B. Gamma emission doesn't change the charge (Z).

70. B. Gamma emission doesn't change the neutron number.

71. C. The "m" stands for metastable.

72. C. This is the definition of an isomeric state.

73. D. The energy of the excited state is emitted as a gamma ray.

74. B. Internal conversion competes with gamma ray emission.

75. A. The energy is internally transferred to the electron which is then emitted.

76. E. The removal of an electron leads to a vacancy in the atomic sheels. This is filled and leads to B or D.

77. A. A β^--particle is an electron.

78. A. Much lighter than

79. D. The neutrino and the β^- share the energy.

80. B. A neutrino carries off part of the energy (Antineutrino is also a correct answer).

81. D. In Z→Z + 1; A→A; 15 + 1 = 16.

82. B. β^--decay changes N→P so N decreases by 1.

83. D. The Z-number is equivalent to the number of protons.

84. D. β^--decay changes A N→P so that Z-number increases by 1.

85. C. The A-number is the same as the number of particles.

86. C. Isobaric decays (β^-, β^+, EC) do not change the number of particles (A number) in the nucleus.

87. B. Electrons (β^-) do not exist in the nucleus; β^--particles are not *atomic* electrons.

88. C. However, this varies quite a bit from nuclide to nuclide. It also varies from 0 to $E_{\beta max}$ for each decay.

89. C. The β^--particles can have any energy from zero up to maximum.

90. A. Positrons have the same mass as electrons but have a positive charge.

91. B. The charge is positive rather than negative.

92. B. The neutrino carries off part of the energy.

93. D. The β^+ and the ν share the energy in a fashion similar to β^--decay.

94. B. Since positron decay changes a proton to a neutron Z→Z−1.

95. A. Since β^+ changes P→N, N increases by 1.

96. C. Changing P→N does not change the A number.

97. C. In β^+-decay the change is P→N.

98. C. In β^+ P→N; Z→Z−1; A→A. So A = 12 and 6 + 1 = 7 = Z.

99. A. The K-shell electron is the one most likely to interact with the nucleus.

100. A. EC changes P→N so N increases by 1.

101. B. Changing P→N leaves the mass number unchanged.

102. C. EC changes P→N so Z decreases by 1.

103. F. Electron capture creates a vacancy in the atomic shells.

104. D. In EC P→N so Z decreases; A stays the same; Z = 31, A = 68.

105. C. An alpha particle is two neutrons and two protons. This is a $^4_2$He nucleus.

106. C. It emits 2 protons (in $^4_2\alpha$-particle), so Z→Z−2.

107. D. It emits 4 particles (nucleons) so A→A−4.

108. B. Z→Z−2; A→A−4 so 226→222 and 88→86.

109. A. This is the definition of a Becquerel.

110. A. This is the definition of a Curie.

111. A. $6 \times 3.7 \times 10^7 = 222 \times 10^6$ Bq = 222 MBq.

112. C. The longer T_p is, the smaller λ is.

113. A. This is the definition of the decay constant.

114. D. $A = A_o e^{-\lambda t}$

115. C. Since it is exponential decay.

116. A. $\lambda = 0.693/Tp = 0.048$; $t = 0.048 \times 3 = 0.145$; $e^{-0.145} = 0.86$; $A = Aoe^{-\lambda t} = 200 \times 0.86 = 173$.

117. B. $\lambda t = 0.335 \times 5 = 1.67$; $e^{-\lambda t} = 0.187$; $A = Aoe^{-\lambda t} = 15 \times 0.187 = 2.8$ mCi.

118. C. 1 week = 168 hr.; $\lambda t = 0.0107 \times 168 = 1.80$ $e^{-\lambda t} = 0.166$; $A = Aoe^{-\lambda t} = 300 \times 0.168 = 50$ μCi

119. A. $\lambda = 0.693/30 = 0.023$; $t = 1$; $e^{-\lambda t} = 0.977$; $A = Aoe^{-\lambda t} = 15 \times 0.977 = 14.7$ mCi.

120. C. $\lambda = 0.693/73 = 0.0095$; $t = 77$ da; $\lambda t = 0.73$ $e^{-\lambda t} = 0.48$; $A = Aoe^{-\lambda t} = 50 \times 0.48 = 24$ μCi.

121. D. $\lambda = 0.693/6 = 0.115$; $t = -7$ hr.; $\lambda t = -0.808$; $e^{-\lambda t} = e^{0.808} = 2.24$; $A = Aoe^{-\lambda t} = 270 \times 2.24 = 606$ mCi.

122. B. $\lambda = 0.693/270 = .0026$; $\lambda t = 0.0026 \times 200 = 0.51$ $e^{-\lambda t} = 0.598$; $A = Aoe^{-\lambda t} = 700 \times 0.598 = 419$ μCi.

123. C. $\lambda t = 1.1$; $e^{-\lambda t} = 0.33$; $\%R = A/A_o = e^{-\lambda t} = 0.33 = 33\%$.

124. B. $\lambda = 0.693/12.4 = 0.056$; $t = -21$ hr; $t = 1.17$ $e^{-\lambda t} = e^{+1.17} = 3.23$; $A = Aoe^{-\lambda t} = 30 \times 3.23 = 97$ μCi.

125. C. $\lambda = 0.693/20.3 = 0.034$; $\%R = A/Ao = e^{-\lambda t}$; $t = 0.034 \times 60 = 2.05$ (time in minutes); $e^{-\lambda t} = 0.129 = 12.9\%$.

126. D. $\lambda = 0.693/64 = 0.0168$; $t = -100$, $\lambda t = 1.08$; $e^{-\lambda t} = 200 \times 2.94 = 589$ μCi.

127. A. $A = Ao\ e^{-\lambda t}$; $t = 0.0069 \times 1440 = 9.9$; (in minutes) $e^{-\lambda t} = 0.000048$; $A = Aoe^{-\lambda t} = 20 \times 0.00048 = 0.00096$ mCi - 0.96 μCi.

128. C. For percent remaining, $\% = e^{-\lambda t} \times 100$, $t = 0.0063 \times 120 = 0.756$ (t must be in minutes) $e^{-\lambda t} = 0.47$.

129. A. $\lambda = 0.693/60 = 0.0116$; $t = 0.24$ (t must be in days); $e^{-\lambda t} = 0.78$; $A = A_o e^{-\lambda t} = 2 \times 0.78 = 1.57$ mCi.

130. C. Here $t = -24$ by . $= 0.693/13 = 0.053$; $t = -1.28$ $e^{-\lambda t} = e^{1.28} = 3.60$; $A = Aoe^{-\lambda t} = 5.6 \times 3.6 = 20$ mCi.

131. A. Gamma -1, Alpha -K = 2.94, from input data.

132. C. Gamma -4 which is emitted 68% of the time (from output data).

133. A. K alpha -1 is emitted 48% of the time.

134. D. Read from the Gamma -2 transition from the input data.

135. B. Read from output data.

136. C. K Alpha -1 x-ray (0.0221).

137. D. The half-life is 2.12×10^5 yr.

138. A. The data are read from the input data.

139. D. The average energy is the mean particle from the output data.

140. C. Average neutrino energy is 1.7100 - 0.6948 = 1.0152.

141. B. β^- decay goes to right; EC and β^+ go to left.

142. B. Mixed since it has both β^- and γ.

143. B. $\lambda = 0.693/Tp = 0.693/4 = 0.17\ hr^{-1}$.

144. A. Since it has long half-life followed by short half-life and emits a single γ-ray of useful energy.

145. D. Since it has a relatively long half-life.

146. C. Three half-lives so 1/8 - 50 mCi.

147. C. β^- changes $N \rightarrow P$.

148. A. β^- changes N→P.

149. A. $^{12}_{6}C$, and $^{14}_{6}C$ have the same Z number.

150. C. $^{133}_{56}Ba$ and $^{133}_{55}Cs$ have the same A number.

151. B. $^{15}_{7}N$ and $^{16}_{8}O$ have 8 neutrons each.

152. D. Co-57 EC

153. D. In-111 EC

154. D. I-125 EC

155. B. I-131 β^-

156. D. Ga-67 EC

157. B. Mo-99 β^-

158. B. P-32 β^-

159. B. Xe-133 β^-

160. C. It takes less than this to create the ions, but this is the average when one counts both the ionization and the excitation.

161. B. This is the definition of LET.

162. B. The alpha particle loses energy faster.

163. B. This is related to the LET.

164. A. $I_1 d_1{}^2 = I_2 d_2{}^2$; $I_2 = I_1 \frac{d_1{}^2}{d_2{}^2} = 50\ (20/45)^2 = 9.9$

165. C. $d_2 = I_1\ I_2\ d = 72{,}000\ 44{,}100\ 18 = 1.28 \times 18^2 = 23$

166. C. $I_1 = I_2\ (d_2/d_1)^2 = 28{,}600\ (14/8)^2 = 87{,}590$

167. B. $t_2 = t_1\ (d_2/d_1)^2 = 1.2(58/15)^2 = 18$ min.

168. B. $I_1 = I_2 (d_2/d_1)^2 = 300 (15/8)^2 = 1055$

169. C. $I_1 = I_2 (d_2/d_1)^2 = 34,000 (3/17)^2 = 1059$

170. D. The mass of the particles is changed to energy. The positrons annihilate with an electron present in the matter. This is an example of $E = mc^2$.

171. B. 2 x 511 = 1022, 511 keV for each photon.

172. C. Positrons always annihilate, have a medium LET, and sometimes produce Bremsstrahlung.

173. B. About 5 mm. Range about 500 mg/cm^2 500/1000 = 0.5 cm.

174. C. This is the definition of Bremsstrahlung.

175. A. The range in air is R (mm) = 3.25 $E^{3/4}$ (MeV). The range in other materials is Rm = 0.00035 Ra Am/βm
Ra = 0.00035 x 3.25 x 18/1 = 0.004 mm.

176. A. Bremsstrahlung production is proportional to Z. The fraction of a beta particle's energy that goes into Bremsstrahlung production is approximately f = ZE/3000 where E is the transition energy in MeV.

177. D. All of these will stop an alpha particle.

178. D. 680 keV = 680,000 eV. 680,000/34 = 20,000.

179. D. All of the energy, minus the binding energy, is transferred to the electron.

180. A. The photon is destroyed in the interaction.

181. C. An Auger electron may also be emitted. The probability depends on the Z number.

182. A. It goes approximately as Z^3.

183. B. The mass coefficient goes as $1/E^3$.

184. A. The K-shell is the one with the highest probability for the interaction.

185. C. Only part of the energy is transferred to the electron.

186. D. The electron energy depends on the angle of scatter.

187. B. The probability of a Compton interaction decreases slowly with time.

188. D. The energy of the scattered photon is minimum for 180 scatter. This is called backscatter.

189. A. Since E/511 increases as E increases.

190. B. This is the mass energy ($E = mc^2$) of the two particles.

191. C. 1.02 MeV is used to create the particles. So the particles share the energy of the photon minus 1.02 MeV.

192. A. The probability of pair production increases with energy. There is a threshold at 1.02 MeV.

193. A. The probability of pair production increases with increasing Z.

194. C. The positron annihilates.

195. C. This is the inverse square law.

196. D. $\mu = 0.693/HVL = 0.693/23.1 = 0.03\ cm^{-1}$

197. C. $200/12.5 = 16.2^4 = 16$; so 4 HVLs.

198. C. $T = I/I_o = e^{-\mu x}$; $x = 0.139 \times 1.2 = 0.167$; $e^{-\mu x} = e^{-0.167} = 0.85$

199. D. $\mu = 0.693/HVL = 0.693/3.85 = 0.18$; $x = 0.18 \times 23 = 4.14$; $T = e^{-\mu x} = e^{-4.14} = 0.016$

200. B. $T = e^{-\mu x}$; $x = 0.45 \times 2 = 0.9$; $e^{-0.9} = 0.41$

201. D. $\mu = 0.693/HVL = 0.693/7.7 = -.09$; $x = 0.09 \times 15 = 1.35$; $T = e^{-\mu x} = e^{-1.35} = 0.26$

202. C. 2 HVLs reduce the intensity to 25%.

203. B. As μ decreases HVL increases 0.693 – ln(2).

204. A. Since there is more material per cm.

205. A. It increases with increasing Z.

206. B. It decreases until pair production becomes predominant.

207. C. It doesn't depend on the speed of the photon.

208. B. Compton scatter predominates at medium energies.

209. A. the photoelectric effect predominates low energy.

210. D. Exponential attenuation A.

211. C. $T = e^{-\mu x}$; $x = 25 \times - .08$ (change mm to cm) $= 2e^{-2} = 0.135$.

212. B. It uses an NaI (T1) crystal.

213. A. Dose calibrators are ionization chambers.

214. A. High count rates overload NaI (Tl) counters.

215. B. This makes it good for measuring the radiation levels around patients.

216. D. The "Cutie Pie" is an ionization chamber.

217. B. They recombine before they can be collected.

218. D. Each ion contributes to the current flow.

219. B. In this region the ions are energetic enough to produce other ions.

220. B. This leads to the gas avalanche.

221. D. Proportional counters are not normally used for clinical counting of radionuclides.

222. A. This lets one insert alpha-sources into the detection chamber.

223. E. Additional ions are created in a gas avalanche. When the ions hit the collection electrode they create Bremsstrahlung, which causes more ions.

224. A. This is the definition of starting potential.

225. B. The quench lowers the voltage and stops the production of Bremsstahlung.

226. B. This can be used as a quality control test.

227. A. This preserves the counter.

228. A. GM counters are more sensitive than "Cutie Pie."

229. A. Scatter changes the amount of radiation that reaches the detector.

230. C. The NaI (Tl) detector is an example.

231. B. It is almost the only scintillator that is used.

232. A. Since it is hygroscopic it must be sealed against moisture.

233. D. The light output is proportional to the energy deposited in the crystal.

234. C. To match the light of the crystal to the PM tube.

235. C. Light from the crystal to an electrical pulse.

236. A. The photons knock the electrons loose and initiate the electrical pulse.

237. B. This is the same photoelectric effect as in the interaction of gamma rays *but* it is created by light photons from the crystal.

238. D. When an electron strikes the crystals it knocks off additional electrons.

239. A. The output is proportional to the energy deposited in the crystal.

240. A. Because of charges in dynode voltage, it doesn't affect B.

241. B. The gain is independent of the energy of gamma ray but depends on the applied voltage. Total gain is about 10 million times.

242. C. Each of these is required for proper signal processing.

243. B. The chief purpose of the preamp is impedance matching.

244. C. Pulse height analyzer.

245. A. A scaler is a pulse counter.

246. B. If the pulse is below the LLD, no pulse is produced. If the pulse is above the LLD but below the ULD, a pulse is produced. If pulse is above LLD and ULD, a pulse is produced by both but cancelled by the anti-coincidence.

247. B. Since it samples for a longer time.

248. A. It has a single photon of medium energy and has a long half-life (30 years).

249. C. Usually the voltage is adjusted. This changes the gain of the photomultiplier tube. On some systems, the fine gain is adjusted.

250. B. This is 20 keV.

251. B. W = 0.15 x 412 = 62 keV, B = 1/2W = 412 - 31 = 381.

252. B. W = 0.15 x 412 = 62 keV, B = 1/2W = 412 - 31 = 381.

253. C. W = 0.10 x 320 = 32 keV, B = E - 1/2W = 320 - 16 = 304.

254. B. W = 0.10 x 320 = 32 keV, B = E - 1/2W = 320 - 16 = 304.

255. C. E = (B + 1/2W) = (240 + 18) = 258.

256. A. The energy is higher so less gain is needed.

257. A. With GR = 1/2 (less gain) each dial setting will be 2 keV so 1050 keV = 525 dial settings.

258. C. Window width is 1400 - 1050 = 350 Gr = 1/2 so window width is 1/2 x 350 = 175 dial setting.

259. B. With the gain of 4 the GR = 414 = 1/2 so each dial setting is 1/2 keV. E = 1/2 (56 + 1/2 12) = 31.

260. D. E = GR (B + 1/2W) = 2&785 + 1/2 25) = 2 (797.5) = 1595.

261. C. The photopeak consists of events that leave all their energy in the crystal.

262. A. This is both photoelectric events and Compton events when the secondary does not escape from the crystal.

263. B. %R = FWHM/PEAK energy = 50/662 = 7.5%.

264. B. The Compton edge.

265. A. This is the scattered radiation that leaves part of its energy in the crystal.

266. B. This is because more secondary radiation would escape from the crystal. This would decrease the number of events in the photopeak and increase the number of events in the Compton scatter distribution.

267. B. This is because of 180° scatter.

268. D. The sum peak occurs when the two x-rays hit the crystal at once.

269. A. This is both common sense and a requirement of the Joint Commission.

270. C. It is less stable when it is warming up, which may take awhile.

271. B. Emission rate in γ-rays/sec. This is the activity in Bq times the number of gamma rays per disintegration.

272. B. The photons that strike the detector.

273. C. It is the area of the detector and the surface area of a sphere centered on the source.

274. D. Efficiency = $(2.5)^2/4 \times 10^2 = 0.0156 = 1.6\%$.

275. D. Efficiency = $(1.5)^2/4 \times 8^2 = 0.0087 = 0.9\%$.

276. B. Less gamma rays will hit the crystal because more will escape the well.

277. B. More of the radioactive material is at a farther distance from the NaI crystal.

278. D. Either A or B works. However, it is usually easier to use method B.

279. D. The square root of the count.

280. B. 68%.

281. C. 95%.

282. D. 99%.

283. A. The square root of 8000 counts is 89 counts.

284. B. The square root of 79,000 counts is 281 counts. To get 2 standard deviations this is multiplied by 2 to yield 562.

285. A. The square root of 54,000 counts is 232 counts.

286. C. The square root of the count rate divided by the time.

287. D. V^2 is the percent value not the fraction. For 5% use 5 not 0.05.

288. C. 40,000/25 = 1600

289. A. The terns are added together.

290. B. The difference between the count rates.

291. C. 58,000/5 - 4000/10 = 11,200 - 400 = 11,200.

292. D. $\sqrt{11{,}600/5 + 400/10} = \sqrt{2320 + 40} = \sqrt{2360} = 48.5.$

293. A. $\sqrt{(10/20) + (5.30)} = \sqrt{0.5 + 0.167} = \sqrt{.667} = 0.82.$

294. C. R = 45 - 30 = 15.

295. A. $\sqrt{(45/10) + (30/15)} = \sqrt{4.5 + 2} = \sqrt{6.5} = 2.5$

296. E.

297. B.

298. C.

299. D.

300. A.

301. B. Dose calibrator is an ionization chamber.

302. B. "Cutie Pie" is an ionization chamber.

303. D. Gas counter is run in GM region.

304. B. Pocket dosimeter is an ionization chamber.

305. F. Well counter is not a gas detector.

306. F. Gamma camera is not a gas detector.

307. B.

308. I.

309. C.

310. D.

311. A.

312. F.

313. E.

314. H.

315. G.

316. C. It increases the area of the dector.

317. A. It stops more of the radiation.

318. E. Efficiency is a ratio.

319. B. They penetrate the crystal better.

320. C. More of the photons hit the crystal.

321. E. If the system is properly calibrated.

322. E. If the system is properly calibrated.

323. T. There are always losses.

324. T. Magnetic fields may cause strange effects in counters.

325. T. The gain is proportional to the gain setting.

326. F. Longer time constants reduce fluctuations.

327. D. The sodium iodide crystal activated with thallium is the best choice because of its efficiency and light output.

328. B. Older gamma cameras have 19 tubes. More recent cameras have between 37 and 91 tubes.

329. B. The electronics determine energy and position.

330. C. Detector efficiency is better for thicker crystals.

331. B. The more energetic gamma rays are more likely to penetrate the crystal without interacting.

332. C. This removes more scatter since scatter is higher on the low side of the peak.

333. B. Because most of the bolus can be in the field of view at one time.

334. B. 10 microseconds.

335. B. About 10 inches.

336. C. About 15 inches.

337. D. The pinhole.

338. A. Thicker collimators hold their resolution better with depth.

339. B. These collimators minimize distortion and give the best trade-off between resolution and efficiency.

340. A. The poorer the resolution of the collimator, the lower its MTF will be.

341. A. The high sensitivity collimator has a faster loss of resolution with depth.

342. B. I/O = f/b = 16/8 = 2. It is magnified by two.

343. A. Increase since the distance decreases.

344. C. This is controlled by the variation in light from event to event.

345. A. The 6-mm (1/4") crystal has the best intrinsic resolution.

346. B. I-131. The intrinsic resolution of the gamma camera is better for higher energy radionuclides.

347. C. Nonlinearities of positrons are the greatest cause of nonuniformity. Nonuniformity of energy response is the second greatest cause.

348. D. So it is often used for first pass cardiac studies.

349. B. Filtered back projection is used.

350. C. Attenuation corrections for SPECT are more difficult than for PET.

351. C. Positron emitters (C-11, N-13, O-15, F-18) are good tags for physiologically active radiopharmaceuticals.

352. B. MTFs are combined by multiplication.

353. A. Efficiency changes as the square of the resolution.

354. B. It is customary to define the byte as 8 bits.

355. C. The number of pixels is found by multiplying the rows and columns of a matrix. 128 x 128 = 16,384.

356. D. The ADC converts analog signals from the computer to digital signals usable by the computer.

357. A. The CPU (the central processing unit) controls the other portions of the computer.

358. B. You need to measure things the same way each time.

359. D. Problems that fix themselves are uncommon.

360. C. The unit must be energy calibrated prior to other tests.

361. B. Plot the data and find the FWHM.

362. B. FWHM/peak energy x 100.

363. B. 61 x 100/662 = 9.2%.

364. A. There are other ways to work this.

365. A. This compares the observed fluctuations to the expected ones.

366. B. Set up a table and calculate χ^2.

367. B. 4.8 is between 4.2 and 8.3.

368. A. Normal counts are 10–90%.

369. C. One needs a large number of counts to reduce statistical fluctuations and a low count rate to avoid dead time effects.

370. A. Scatter from the collimator can shift the apparent photopeak to a lower energy level. However, in newer cameras the difference is small and convenience may dictate leaving it on.

371. C. Changing the intensity affects the dot focus so the dots should be focused each time the intensity is changed.

372. D. If the source is nonuniform it must be returned to the manufacturer; if it has high energy contamination it can be aged for several months.

373. D. Dirty rollers cause film jams and irregular development; dirt on lenses lowers image quality.

374. B. LSF is a measure of spatial resolution.

375. A. This is the most important test of γ-camera performance.

376. B. Interaction of radiation with the cellular component is nonpreferential probability function which may or may not result in damage.

377. D. Purine and pyrimidine sequence can be changed by radiation. The weak hydrogen bond which links the two DNA chains is easily broken.

378. C. The cell contains many entities of variable radiosensitivity, but those located in the nucleus are most sensitive.

379. E. Increasing number of cells will be killed with an increase in radiation dose.

380. C. Inhibition of cell division which ultimately leads to death is called "reproductive death."

381. D. In addition to the above, radiation may induce changes in protein solubility and destruction of individual amino acids.

382. C. Radiation sensitivity is a function of the cell's mitotic activity; the higher the rate, the higher radiosensitivity. The small lymphocyte is a notable exception.

383. A. Cells that are not specialized for a specific function are more radiosensitive than the highly specialized cells.

384. A. LET is the rate at which an ionizing event loses energy per length of track and is expressed as keV/micron.

385. B. In contrast to electromagnetic radiation, highly ionizing particulate radiation like alpha particles and neutrons have high LET.

386. A. Although certain chemicals, some viruses, and ultraviolet light can produce mutations, radiation is a most effective method for producing mutations.

387. D. A certain number of spontaneous mutations is produced with each increment increase in radiation dose. Mutation frequency is dose dependent, but dose-rate independent.

388. C. Most radiation-induced mutations are harmful, and because most of them are also recessive, they can be retained for generations. Mutations of dominant genes are eliminated more quickly by natural selection.

389. B. Mutations are defined as permanent alterations in the sequence of purine and pyrimidine bases on the DNA molecule, or in the amount or volume of DNA.

390. D. Frequency of mutations increases linearly with dose of radiation and even very small doses can result in mutations.

391. A. Alteration of the genetic material may manifest itself as a mutation.

392. C. Carcinogesis of leukemia is believed to have a latent period of 5 to 8 years.

393. B. The latent period of leukemia is thought to be 5 to 8 years, and 15 years for other types of malignancies.

394. B. The frequency of radiation-induced mutations increases linearly with dose, with no known threshold dose below which mutations could not be induced.

395. B. Radiations that are more densely ionizing (efficient in producing high numbers of ion pairs), such as alpha particles, have been shown to produce large number of mutations.

396. D. Latent period is free of overt manifestations of radiation damage.

397. B. Decreased life span in irradiated humans may be due to nonspecific causes, i.e., other than radiation-induced malignant disease.

398. C. The $LD_{50/30}$ concept is usually applied when studying the effects of acute radiation lethality in mammals.

399. A. Although the estimated $LD_{50/30}$ varies with source, it is believed to range from 250 to 450 rads.

400. D. Other factors which can influence response to radiation are: sex, environmental factors, presence of radiation sensitizers or protectors, and individual response.

401. D. $$\text{RBE} = \frac{\text{Dose (rads) from 250 keV x-ray to achieve same effect}}{\text{Dose (rads) from another radiation needed to achieve the same effect.}}$$

402. A. Fast neutrons, protons, and alpha particles are 10 times as damaging as x- and gamma rays.

403. B. Increased radiation response in presence of oxygen (oxygen effect) has been well documented in many biological systems, both in vivo and in vitro.

404. C. Partial recovery due to repair of biologic damage will occur between the periods of irradiation.

405. D. Nausea, vomiting, and diarrhea are referred to collectively as the NVD syndrome. Additionally, the level of circulating leukocytes will frequently increase with a concomitant decrease in lymphocytes.

406. A. Initial period of response to an acute total-body radiation exposure is characterized by nausea, vomiting, and diarrhea.

407. C. Reproductive death or failure is defined as the inability of a cell to undergo repeated mitoses after irradiation.

408. B. Extensive destructive changes in the histology of the intestinal mucosa are believed to be responsible for early (3 to 5 days) death in animals exposed to 900 to 10,000 rads of x- or gamma rays.

409. D. Changes seen in brain and the spinal cord following 10,000 rads of x- or gamma radiation are consistent with the signs and symptoms manifested by irradiated animals.

410. A. Radiation-induced gut damage does not become manifest for several days, a patient with CNS syndrome dies before gut damage becomes apparent.

411. B. Radiation sickness, or total body radiation syndrome, by definition, results from an acute, whole-body (or nearly whole-body) exposure to external penetrating radiation such as x-, gamma rays, or neutrons.

412. C. The total dose of whole-body irradiation largely determines the severity of response.

413. B. Although fractionated exposure of the whole body may result in signs and symptoms of the GI syndrome, true syndrome, by definition, requires an acute, one-time exposure of the whole body (or nearly the whole body).

414. D. Dose of radiation necessary to produce a true GI syndrome will most seriously compromise the bone marrow and its ability to repopulate depleted levels of circulating white blood cells.

415. D. Exposure to high dose of radiation may seriously compromise or inhibit the ability of bone marrow to maintain sufficient number of circulating red and white cells.

416. B. Bone marrow, lymph organs, intestines, testes are all very sensitive to irradiation.

417. B. Although the lymphocyte does not divide and should be radioresistant, it is, in fact, exceedingly radiosensitive.

418. D. Blood stem cells are highly radiosensitive. Radiation inhibits their mitosis either by outright destruction or by interfering with normal nuclear function.

419. B. Genetic mutations and damage to somatic cells may not be overtly expressed until years or generations after exposure.

420. C. Although it is not the only carcinogen, radiation has been shown to produce malignancy in nearly all tissues and animals tested.

421. A. Exposure to diagnostic (small) doses of x-rays during the first 2 weeks of pregnancy may result in gross fetal abnormalities and abortion.

422. D. The period of organogenesis is characterized by very high rate of mitosis and initial differentiation of the cells. Death of the embryo may be secondary to anatomical abnormalities.

423. A. Because of the high incidence of gross fetal abnormalities, some authorities feel that therapeutic abortion is justified if the fetus has been exposed to a radiation dose of 10 rads or more.

424. B. The early embryo is exquisitely sensitive to ionizing radiation during preimplantation phase and during organogenesis.

425. D. In addition to the above, microphthalmia, strabismus, hydrocele, mongolism, spina bifida, blindness, limb deformities, etc. have been observed.

426. A. A therapeutic dose of 5 mCi of I^{131} taken orally will result in chromosome aberrations in lymphocytes, and can produce sterility in the human female.

427. B. Administration of radionuclides to gravid animals has resulted in fetal abnormalities and death.

428. D. The length of exposure and radiosensitivity of the adjacent tissue would also be a factor in the amount of damage.

429. C. No statement.

430. A. Factors such as the amount of radionuclides in the total body, the amount of radionuclides in the organ of interest, the mass of the organ and the rate of radionuclide uptake by the organ, are only some of the factors which must be determined before internal dose calculations can be made.

431. B. Alpha and beta particles are considered to be radiations with high LET, and while their penetrability is limited, they are capable of producing serious lesions in their immediate proximity.

432. A. Physical and biological half-lives are included in calculation of radionuclide's effective half-life.

433. A. Biological half-life is the time required for one-half of the radionuclide to be excreted by the body.

434. B. The technologist should also know how to detect and measure the radionuclide, the means for his (and his patient's) protection, and the procedure for safe disposal of all contaminated materials.

435. B. This figure does not include medical radiation. The principal sources are external (cosmic radiation from space and gamma rays from earth's crust), and internal (ingested), consisting mainly of potassium and carbon. The average annual medical dose to an individual is about 20 mrem, consisting mostly of radiation used in diagnostic procedures.

436. A. Effects of background radiation, genetic effects, and occupational exposure may mask the hazards which could be attributed to medical exposure. It is not possible to distinguish the effects of low level background and medical radiation.

437. D. There is no known dose below which damage may not occur. For this reason all possible precautions must always be taken to keep the radiation dose to the patient and the technologist as low as reasonably possible.

438. B. The benefit of medical radiation almost always clearly prevails even when very large (therapeutic) doses are considered.

439. A. Although radiation is a known carcinogen, and induction of new malignancies within or outside the treatment area may occur, such occurrence is known to happen in less than 1% of the patients treated with therapeutic doses of radiation.

440. D. Because the radioactivity is usually administered internally in nuclear medicine procedures, evaluation of risk presents a new set of problems. Some of the factors to be considered include radionuclide's physical, chemical, and biological properties, critical organ, and presence of pathology.

441. A. Elimination of beta emitters, selective blocking of noncritical organs not under study, use of efficient counting and storage equipment, and "doing it right the first time" will reduce the patient's radiation dose (and its inherent risk).

442. C. Diagnostic ultrasound, usually used at 1 to 15 MHz frequency, has not shown adverse effects. Because human studies have been few, deleterious effects cannot be ruled out. Ultrasound at levels far above diagnostic levels can produce significant heat and hyperthermia. Compared to procedures which employ ionizing radiation, ultrasound is considered to be relatively safe, but its use should be considered on a risk vs benefit basis.

443. C. Cavitation is a normal attenuation process for ultrasound. It results in growth of gas bubbles present in all fluids. Absorption of sound energy also occurs by formation of heat, and by another direct process which is not understood.

444. B. It measures total exposure.

445. C. Defined for x- and gamma rays *only*.

446. C. It is charge liberated in air by radiation.

447. B. The f-factor converts roentgens to rads. The f-factor is about one for soft tissue.

448. D. REM is always defined.

449. B. REM = RADS X RBE. RBE is 1 for radiations used in nuclear medicine.

450. B. RBE for 140 gamma rays = 1.

451. B. QF for ^{32}P beta-particles = 1.

452. C. QF for alpha-particles > 1.

453. C. A 100 rads is 1 gray.

454. C. 50 Gray or 5000 rem.

455. D. The Sievert is 100 REMs.

456. C. Sieverts = Gray x QF.

457. B. The same as the whole body.

458. B. The same as for the whole body.

459. D. In a well-run department the dose to a technologist should be very low. The technologist should not be involved in high-risk procedures such as radionuclide therapy.

460. A. The dose rate near the patients can be high. Although it is unlikely that the nurse will exceed 0.5 rem, it is desirable to keep the exposure as low as possible.

461. A. Because the nurse may spend a long time near that patient.

462. B. 5 rem.

463. A. It excludes all natural sources such as internal radiation, cosmic rays, and external background.

464. D. 0.5 rem or 500 mrem.

465. B. 0.5 rem, the same as a nonradiation worker.

466. C. 75 rem to the hands.

467. B. 5 rem per year.

468. B. 5 rem.

469. B. They are like everyone in the general population.

470. B. 18.

471. D. This dose is to a small volume.

472. B. "Well-run" are the key words. In a poor laboratory you can receive radiation from A, B, C, and D.

473. D. Most comes from imaging.

474. B. Shields should always be used.

475. B. (75,000/(50 weeks x 5 days)) = 300 mR/day
300/20,000 = 0.015 hr 1 min.

476. D. This has been measured.

477. C. One meter.

478. C. So a person 20 years of age could have an accumulated dose of 10 rem.

479. B. 50 rem.

480. A. 5 rem. Although the lifetime accumulated dose is 100 rem, the maximum dose for any one year should not exceed 5 rem. The most that is permitted is 3 rem per quarter.

481. A. B, C, and D must be specified.

482. C. 30 mCi

483. T. On two surfaces.

484. T. 10 mR/hr

485. F. There should be no eating or drinking anywhere there is radioactivity.

486. T. Since the hands may receive a large exposure.

487. F. Badges are not sensitive enough to change weekly.

488. T. Since the activity is low.

489. F. Because of the possibility of contamination.

490. T. To protect against internal contamination.

491. T. To protect against hand contamination.

492. F. To prevent contamination.

493. T. Since he may contaminate them.

494. F. This increases the risk of contamination.

495. F. It is unlikely they will be contaminated.

496. T. Because of the inverse square law.

497. A. The two lighter nuclei fuse to form a heavier nucleus. Energy is released in the process.

498. C. This is the definition of fission.

499. A. Spontaneous is natural, induced is by neutron bombardment.

500. A. Neutrons.

501. B. Fission is the splitting of large nuclei to make lighter ones.

502. C. Uranium and plutonium.

503. A. Isotope.

504. C. Such as the ^{99}Mo—^{99m}Tc generator.

505. D. An alumina ion exchange column will bind Mo-99 but not Tc-99m. When the generator is elected the Mo stays bound to the column and the Tc washes out.

506. C. Alumina column.

507. D. Since the activity of the Mo-99 changes during the time of observation.

508. C. TcO_4^- is pertechnetate.

509. B. The Tc must be reduced to facilitate binding.

510. C. If the generator is not working properly Mo-99 breakthrough can occur with any elution.

511. B. No more than 1 μCi of Mo-99 per 1 mCi of Tc-99m.

512. C. No more than 5 μCi of Mo-99 per dose of Tc-99m.

513. A. (15/200). 50 = 3.75 μCi of ^{99}Mo. This is less than 5 so it can be used.

514. B. By 3:00 p.m. (7 hr.) the Tc has decayed to 89 mCi (15/89) .50 = 8.4 μCi. This is over the 5 μCi limit.

515. B. 20 ug/ml for reaction, 10 ug/ml for fission.

516. C. Radiochemical refers to the chemical form of the substance.

517. B. Radionuclide refers to the nuclide in the substance.

518. B. The ^{99}Mo is an undesirable radionuclide when it is mixed with Tc-99m.

519. C. The free ^{131}I is not the desired chemical form.

520. B. Concentration is activity per unit volume (usually in ml).

521. B. 250/5 = 50.

522. C. This is the C = A/V equation rearranged.

523. D. 15/58 = 0.26.

524. D. 350/30 = 11.67.

525. B. 385/3 = 128.

526. C. 100/128 = 0.78.

527. A. 23/11.67 = 1.97.

528. B. Vol = 100 + 10, C = 18/110 = 0.164 mCi - 164 μCi.

529. A. The 10 ml that are removed are 10% of the 100 ml.

530. D. 5% of 50 = 0.05 x 50 = 2.5 ml.

531. B. This is the method that uses the concentration of the radioactivity, the energy emitted by the radionuclide and the absorbed fraction to calculate the dose.

532. D. All the factors are used.

533. B. 70 kg is a standard man.

534. C. Since all the energy tha is emitted is absorbed in the target organ, the absorbed fraction is 100% (1).

535. C. The excretion is biological and does not have anything to do with whether it is radioactive.

536. A. This comes from $\frac{1}{T_e} = \frac{1}{T_p} + \frac{1}{T_b}$

$$\frac{1}{T_e} = \frac{T_b + T_p}{T_b \times T_p}; \quad Te = \frac{T_p \times T_b}{T_p + T_b}$$

537. It can not be longer than the shorter of either the physical or the biological.

538. D. $T_b = \frac{T_b \times T_e}{T_b - T_e} = \frac{26 \times 18}{26 - 18} = 468/18 = 58.5 = 59$

539. B. $T_b = \frac{T_p \times T_e}{T_p = T_e} = \frac{6 \times 2.4}{6 - 2.4} = 14.4/2.6 = 4$

540. A. $T_e = \frac{T_p \times T_b}{T_p + T_b} = \frac{8 \times 6}{8 + 6} = 48/14 = 3.4$

541. B. $T_e = \frac{T_p \times T_b}{T_p + T_b} = \frac{1/4 \times 6}{1/4 + 6} = 1.5/6.25 = 0.24 \text{ hr} = 14.4 \text{ min.}$

542. C. The target.

543. A. Bombarded by radiation.

544. B. B which produces radiation.

545. D. C and product nucleus D.

546. D. The plasma proteins are usually divided into albumin, globulin, and fibrinogen, which comprise respectively 4.8%, 2.3%, and 0.3% of the plasma. Hormones are transported by certain globulin fractions.

547. A. Hemoglobin plays a role in oxygen and CO_2 transport as well as regulation of blood pH.

548. A. Conversely, the fluid portion of coagulated blood is known as serum.

549. D. After approximately 120 days, the red cells are destroyed by the RE system, and the hemoglobin released.

550. D. Approximately 65% of the total body stores of iron is present in the form of hemoglobin.

551. A. Thrombocytes is another name for platelets, which take part in blood coagulation.

552. D. Themain function of granulocytes is to combat infections.

553. D. Fibrinogen in the plasma is converted into strands of fibrin by the action of the enzyme thrombin.

554. C. They also participate in the processes of blood coagulation and clot retraction.

555. C. The volume of the plasma is then called the plasmacrit.

556. C. Hematocrits normally average 45%, with the plasmacrit at 55% normally.

557. C. Serum, unlike plasma, contains no fibrinogen.

558. B. The grayish-colored layer of cells just above the red cells is the white cell population.

559. A. Hematocrit determinations are performed on anticoagulated blood and measure the ratio between the plasma and the packed red cells in a spun sample.

560. A. Dehydration causes the plasma volume to decrease. Since the hematocrit is a ratio between plasma and packed cells, the packed cell portion will appear greater with a decrease in the plasma portion.

561. B. The dilution principle uses the equation $Q = VC$, where Q is the total quantity of tracer, V is the diluting volume, and C is the tracer concentration.

562. A. In this equation, Q equals the quantity of tracer, V is the diluting volume, and C is the tracer concentration in diluting fluid.

563. A. The geometric efficiency of the well counter is such that lower energy nuclides may be used, thus keeping patient exposure at an acceptable level.

564. D. Both red cells or plasma can easily be labeled with a radioactive marker for blood volume tests.

565. F. RCV is also useful in pre-op and post-op evaluations, hypotension, and in cases of extensive trauma and burns.

566. D. The normal adult male should have a total blood volume of 72 ml/kg, while the normal adult female should have 66 ml/kg.

567. D. ^{51}Cr sodium chromate.

568. C. ^{51}Cr has a gamma energy of 320 keV and a physical half-life of 27.8 days.

569. C. Hexavalent chromium can permeate the red cell membrane. The addition of ascorbic acid during the labeling procedure reduces the chromium to the trivalent state, which can't penetrate the red cell membrane.

570. E. The rate of binding of chromate to RBCs is accelerated by increasing temperatures and acidity.

571. D. Both antibiotics and polyvitamins will reduce the hexavalent chromium to a trivalent state before it can tag the red cells in the standard whole blood.

572. D. ACD (acid citrate dextrose) solution acts as an anticoagulant for the whole blood while in vitro tagging with the radiotracer takes place.

573. C. ACD solution, with a pH of approximately 6.5, should not exceed the 1:5 ratio to whole blood as excess ACD may cause red cell damage.

574. C. Dextrose acts as a reducing agent in ACD solution.

575. D. Trivalent chromium will not permeate the red cell membrane. Therefore, tagging ceases with the addition of ascorbic acid.

576. B. Extravasation of the dose and excessive binding of the ^{51}Cr by leukocytes or platelets also cause falsely elevated results.

577. F. All of the choices will damage the red cells in a sample.

578. D. A portion of the tracer tends to adhere to the vessel wall at the site of injection, which would tend to erroneously increase counts in a sample taken at that site.

579. B. Radiolabels used in circulating blood volume must be completely, rapidly, and uniformly distributed throughout the circulatory system.

580. F. In these cases, to ensure that proper mixing has occurred, serial samples should be taken until there is no significant difference in their counts.

581. A. Extravasation of the dose results in the entire dose not being injected into the vein, with falsely low counts coming from the subsequent samples. Further calculations result in falsely high blood volume results.

582. D. The average whole body hematocrit is roughly 92% of the venous blood hematocrit. This discrepancy occurs because of the differences in the hematocrits of blood obtained from different sized vessels as well as from different organs. In addition, plasma trapped in cells can introduce a 2-4% error in hematocrit values.

583. A. The use of Group O, Rh^- blood is one modification in measuring blood volume.

584. D. High levels of background activity from previously administered radionuclides will yield falsely low values in a red cell volume.

585. B. Normal adult male plasma volumes average approximately 44 ml/kg of body weight.

586. D. Radioiodinated ^{125}I human serum albumin is most commonly utilized for plasma volume determinations.

587. C. ^{51}Cr sodium chromate tags to the beta chain of the hemoglobin molecule in the red blood cell.

588. A. Plasma volume determinations are based on the ability to label the plasma component of the blood with a radionuclide.

589. D. ^{125}I has a gamma energy of 35 keV and a physical half-life of 60 days.

590. B. Protein-bound tracers such as ^{125}I albumin (RISA) transfer in and out of the vascular/extravascular beds in the same manner as untagged proteins.

591. E. Exercise and cold weather conditions tend to decrease the plasma volume, while warm climates and pregnancy will increase the normal plasma volume.

592. B. This is much shorter than expected. A major part of this difference is due to the elution of the ^{51}Cr from intact surviving cells (approximately 1%/day).

593. C. Percents are plotted on the log scale, time lapse in days on the linear scale, and a line is drawn through 50% to determine survival half-time.

594. F. For cohort labeling, ^{59}Fe ferrous citrate is used in which the reticulocytes incorporate the radioiron, which then reappears in the circulation as new red blood cells.

595. A. During this same interval, any injected plasma radioactivity is cleared from the circulation.

596. B. Hematocrit readings are taken as the samples come in, but counting of samples is done simultaneously at the conclusion of the study.

597. C. Counting the samples as they are collected will introduce erroneously high count rates toward the beginning of the study, tapering off toward the end.

598. B. Cells labeled by the cohort method are all of the same age since labeling takes place at the site of erythropoiesis.

599. C. In the selective labeling technique for determination of red cell survival, all of the labeled cells are of the same age. They are monitored for their entire life span.

600. D. Cohort or selective labeling follows the life span of the erythrocyte from its origin to its destruction, which normally takes approximately 120 days. This necessitates sampling for up to 4 months in some cases.

601. C. On the other hand, intracorpuscular defects can only be detected using the patient's own cells.

602. F. Blood transfusions and acute blood loss occurring during the red cell survival study will cause an artificially shortened half-time.

603. E. Hypersplenism and hemolytic anemia result in increased rate of destruction of RBCs and thus shortened survival times.

604. D. The red cell survival time will be erroneously shortened in all these conditions.

605. F. All of these studies use ^{51}Chromium (sodium chromate) as the label. Its 320 keV energy prohibits dosages necessary for scintigraphy.

606. B. This study is usually performed in conjunction with the red cell survival study on patients who have evidence of increased red cell destruction.

607. C. Precordium counts represent blood activity, while the liver and spleen represent areas where damaged and sensecent RBCs are sequestered for breakdown.

608. A. With splenic enlargement, either by passive congestion or active disease, the splenic ratio increases.

609. D. Total body iron pool is 5 gm. Three grams of iron is thought to be incorporated into hemoglobin, 1.5 gm is in storage (ferritin and hemosiderin), and 0.5 gm is involved in metabolic activities other than erythropoiesis.

610. C. Total body iron content ranges from 2 to 6 gm and tends to remain fixed within narrow limits.

611. C. This amount lost must be closely matched by absorption through dietary routes.

612. C. The rate and degree of iron absorption depend on the state of the iron stores, degree of hematopoietic activity, and the dietary iron intake.

613. C. Transferrin is the normal iron-transport protein found in the plasma.

614. B. Normal patients with adequate iron reserves will show a plasma iron clearance time of 1-2 hours.

615. D. All half-time determinations are usually plotted on semilogarithmic graph paper.

616. F. These conditions often produce a plasma iron clearance rate (PICR) of less than 60 minutes. PICR are prolonged in conditions such as aplastic anemia and hemochromatosis.

617. C. Pernicious anemia and hemochromatosis will also result in a prolonged plasma iron turnover rate (PITR).

618. C. The PITR can be used as an index of total erythropoietic activity.

619. E. Iron-deficiency anemia and blood loss will also cause the iron utilization rates to accelerate.

620. C. The time for the injected radioiron to be incorporated within RBCs and released into the circulation can be used as an indicator of bone marrow function.

621. B. Anticoagulants such as EDTA and sodium citrate will chelate the radioiron and remove it from circulation via urinary excretion.

622. D. As in splenic sequestration studies, counts are taken over the liver, spleen, and precordium. In addition, sacrum counts are taken to represent marrow erythropoietic activity.

623. D. ^{52}Fe has also been utilized, but is not readily available.

624. C. Utilization rates will be high in polycythemia vera and iron deficiency anemia. Pernicious anemia and hypoplastic anemia result in low utilization rates.

625. A. A peak in activity over the sacrum represents uptake in the bone marrow; the decrease in activity which follows represents the release of RBCs labeled with the radioiron into the circulation.

626. C. After the increase in counts over the sacral area representing bone marrow activity, newly formed erythrocytes containing radioiron are released into the general circulation, eliciting peak counts over the precordium.

627. B. Shorter spans are indicative of conditions such as hemolytic anemias, while ineffective erythropoiesis causes prolonged times.

628. D. A deficiency in intrinsic factor may be caused by pernicious anemia, total or subtotal gastrectomy, or a congenital abnormality.

629. B. The stomach's parietal cells secrete intrinsic factor.

630. D. The stomach's parietal cells produce the protein, intrinsic factor, which renders vitamin B_{12} absorbable by the terminal ileum.

631. F. Vitamin B_{12} is essential for proper functioning of all tissues; however, the GI tract, nervous system, and erythropoietic activity of the bone marrow are most profoundly affected.

632. D. Additionally, vitamin B_{12} deficiency may be the result of gastrointestinal surgery, such as gastrectomy.

633. A. The classic vitamin B_{12} deficiency syndrome is pernicious anemia, which results from a deficiency of the gastric secretion of intrinsic factor.

634. A. Urine is the primary route of excretion. In an abnormal state where malabsorption occurs, fecal excretion occurs.

635. E. In addition, whole-body radioactivity counting has also been utilized.

636. D. Other tests which determine the extent of vitamin B_{12} absorption include fecal excretion and hepatic uptake of the vitamin. Plasma radioactivity test has also been used.

637. B. In addition, if the patient is to have serum B_{12} level done, this should be collected prior to starting the test.

638. D. Administration of ACTH is also an interfering factor. A fasting state is a desirable preparation of the Schilling test to allow the radioactive B_{12} to bind to intrinsic factor.

639. B. The flushing dose of vitamin B_{12} is given approximately 2 hours after ingestion of the radioactive B_{12}.

640. B. The nonradioactive B_{12} serves to "flush" out much of the radioactive B_{12} in the body before it binds to the plasma protein, transcobalomin. Excretion is via the urine, where it can be measured.

641. B. The labeled B_{12} will not be flushed out effectively, resulting in a falsely low value.

642. A. In addition, the amount of "cold" vitamin B_{12} given should be in the range of 0.25-2 μg, a quantity similar to one that might be found in a normal meal. Quantities exceeding this range may not represent normal absorption pathways.

643. A. Normalization of the result after intrinsic factor denotes that the impaired absorption of B_{12} is caused by lack of adequate secretion of intrinsic factor.

644. D. 5% is a low value and may also be indicative of Zollinger-Ellison disease, drug therapy, and genetic abnormalities.

645. D. Pernicious anemia is caused by a deficiency in the gastric production of intrinsic factor. Therefore, administration of intrinsic factor should correct the condition. No improvement in the percent excreted with the addition of intrinsic factor indicates a defect in the intestinal tract.

646. B. Since the energies of ^{57}Co and ^{58}Co (122 keV, 810 keV respectively) are so disparate, differentiation by gamma spectroscopy is possible.

647. C. Intrinsic factor deficiency responds positively when the Schilling test is repeated with a concurrent administration of the hog intrinsic factor. Failure to increase urinary excretion of tagged vitamin B_{12} in this manner may be indicative of parasitic and/or bacterial competition for the vitamin.

648. C. Accurate results of the test demand meticulous collection of the 24-hour urine samples.

649. E. Radiocolloid particles are used to visualize the RE portion, while isotopes of iron are generally used to image the erythroid marrow.

650. E. In addition, bone marrow scanning can assist in localization of biopsy sites, extent of hypertrophies in marrow distribution as in polycythemia vera, and in determining sites for transplants.

651. B. Radiocolloids are used to visualize the reticuloendothelial cells of the marrow, while radioiron images the erythroid portion. ^{51}Cr sodium chromate binds to formed red blood cells.

652. A. In patients with chronic hemolytic anemia, extension of active marrow may occur distally into the long bones and the skull. Note that in pediatric patients, long bone extension of marrow activity is a normal variant.

653. D. Acute hemolytic anemia will image as a normal marrow scan pattern, in contrast to its chronic counterpart, which shows a marked peripheral expansion of bone marrow.

654. D. In addition, bone marrow scanning is useful in assessing the chronicity of anemias, radiation effects, and myelofibrosis.

655. C. Compared to the radioiron agents used to image the bone marrow, ^{99m}Tc sulfur colloid is easily prepared and widely available. Despite its apparent drawbacks, it is still the agent of choice in initial attempts to image the bone marrow.

656. A. The rate of this loss averages about 10% per hour, which makes it negligible within 15 minutes of the test.

657. A. ^{32}P diisopropyl fluorophosphate as an in vivo label is also used in platelet survival studies.

658. A. In addition to measuring the survival time by sampling, external counting has also been helpful in the determination of sites of platelet sequestration, as in thrombocytopenia purpura.

659. D. Other radiopharmaceuticals which have been employed in white cell survival studies are ^{32}P phosphate and diisopropyl fluorophosphate, ^{3}H thymidine. Lymphocytes can be labeled using ^{67}Ga, ^{197}Hg, and ^{99m}Tc.

660. C. Red cell survival is also used to evaluate the effectiveness of therapy of patients with hemolytic anemia.

661. B. When the radioactivity has fallen to half of its original value, the study is generally terminated and the survival half-time calculated.

662. D. The amount of radioactive antigen-antibody complex formed can then be counted and extrapolated from the curve.

663. D. Other terms encompassed by the broad term RIA include radiostereoassay, radioenzymatic assay, and competitive inhibition.

664. C. The basic radioimmune reaction consists of labeled antigen competing physiochemically with an unlabeled antigen for binding sites on a specific antibody. Some hepatitis marker RIAs use labeled antibody instead of labeled antigen.

665. A. Le Chatelier's principle is the third property of equilibrium and refers to the ability of a system to maintain equilibrium despite perturbations such as temperature, pH, and ionic strength.

666. B. Antibodies are produced in response to invasion by foreign substances in the body known as antigens.

667. C. In radioimmunoassay, the term antigen is synonymous with both immunogen and ligand. Antibody and antisera are also synonymous. A hapten can be made antigenic by coupling with a larger molecule.

668. A. Substances with molecular weights of less than 5000 must be covalently coupled to a larger molecule, such as a protein, in order to induce an immunologic response.

669. A. The most common adjuvant used to produce antibodies for RIA procedures is Freund's adjuvant, which is composed of a neutral detergent, mineral oil, and killed bacteria.

670. C. Titer is defined as the optimal or final concentration of the antibody in the assay system.

671. A. The most important consideration would be that antibody's affinity for the antigen of interest. Titer and quantity of antibody produced is of course important, but it must be specific to be useful. As for the source, horse, goat, and rabbit antisera have all been used as sources of antisera according to the particular system under study.

672. C. The higher the affinity of the antibody for the ligand, the higher the sensitivity.

673. F. A radiolabeled antigen with an unimpaired reactivity with the antibody is one of the essential components of any radioimmunoassay system.

674. D. The higher the concentration of the unlabeled antigen (amount in patient's sample), the fewer the antibody reaction sites available for the labeled antigen, resulting in a lower amount of labeled antibody-antigen complex being formed.

675. C. Accuracy and precision are closely related, but precision refers specifically to reproducibility.

676. B. Specificity and selectivity refer to the same concept—the reactor substance must measure or select only one substance among thousands present in a biologic fluid.

677. D. When both avidity and affinity are high, the equilibrium constant is also large. Therefore, a smaller concentration of ligand is needed to saturate the SRS-binding sites, and the more sensitive the system is to small amounts of ligand.

678. E. Antibodies, which are a group of serum proteins, are also known as gamma globulins.

679. D. Ligands can be substances such as hormones, drugs, tumor markers, viruses, and bacteria for which measurement of such in the body is desired. Antibodies, immunoglobulins, and specific reactor substance are terms used interchangeably to mean the component in the radioimmune reaction which binds specifically with the labeled and unlabeled forms of the ligand, thus allowing measurement.

680. D. Nonspecific binding tubes demonstrate degrees of cross-reactivity and specificity.

681. D. The standard curve is derived from the counts coming from the tubes with known concentrations, namely the standards.

682. A. 10^{-12} gm is equal to one picogram, which is the amount which most RIAs can detect.

683. D. The disadvantages of RIA arise mainly from instability of the reagents, lack of reference standards, physiologic factors, and methodologic differences.

684. B. In cases when sensitivity is less important, room temperature incubation is adequate. However, the reproducibility and precision of an assay improve with extended incubations in a cold environment.

685. D. These three components are interdependent, and suboptimal concentration of any one produces a nonacceptable curve.

686. C. The equilibrium or association constant, also known as K, is expressed mathematically as the products involved in the chemical reaction divided by the reactants.

687. C. While ^{131}I, used in the earlier RIA procedures, has a higher specific activity than ^{125}I, it forms a less stable compound due to the presence of beta radiation. In addition, its 8-day half-life is not adequate.

688. D. In addition, the presence of various contaminants which interfere with or degrade a reactive portion of the assay molecule will affect the equilibrium constant, K.

689. B. Parallelism in an assay indicates that diluted sera will provide accurate test results, particularly in cases where a sample has concentrations above the highest standard on the standard curve.

690. A. Recovery of the analyte, which reflects accuracy of the kit, can also be determined by dividing the total analyte recovered by the total analyte added.

691. B. This requirement makes RIA procedures more desirable than many other assay procedures.

692. A. The percent coefficient of variation (% cv) is calculated by dividing the standard deviation by the mean of a series of identical samples.

693. B. Cross-reactivity can occur between different hormones of the same species such as FSH, LH, TSH, and HGH. Cross-reacting antibodies can be minimized by purification techniques similar to the affinity-chromatography purification process.

694. B. Water-soluble carbodiimide can be used to couple hapten derivatives with free amino acid groups to the carboxyl group of a protein.

695. D. ^{125}I is currently the radiolabel of choice for use in RIA procedures.

696. B. After the reactants in the radioimmune reaction have reacted for the specified period of time, a method to separate the bound and free portions must be used in order to measure one or the other segment. All of the methods listed in the statement have been used for this purpose.

697. C. Lactoperoxidase is used in radioiodination procedures and involves oxidation of the iodide.

698. D. Sephadex columns are used as a type of gel filtration separation.

699. A. Gel filtration methods are slow and not applicable to a large number of samples; therefore, they are not used extensively.

700. C. This method involves precipitation of the bound antibody-analyte complex by a second antiserum, an anti-gamma globulin.

701. E. Linear-linear scales will produce a curved dose-response curve, while log-linear and log-logit scales both produce a straight line.

702. C. The Scatchard plot is the classic method for estimating the equilibrium constant, K, which in turn enables component concentration to allow knowledge of optimal sensitivity.

703. C. The zona glomerulosa, zona fasciculata, and the zona reticularis are the three parts of the adrenal cortex. The glomerulosa secretes aldosterone, the fasciculata secretes cortisol, and the reticularis secretes various estrogens and androgens.

704. B. ACTH, or adrenocorticotropic hormone, directly controls the rate of cortisol secretion. Its secretion, in turn, is controlled by the corticotropin-releasing factor from the hypothalamus in a negative feedback fashion.

705. A. There is an overall diurnal variation in the secretion of ACTH and thus cortisol whereby the main secretory phase occurs during the last 3 hours of sleep and first waking hour and decreases to a minimum at night.

706. B. Hypoglycemia, along with pain, trauma, hemorrhage, febrile reactions, and stress, can all cause stimulation of the pituitary-adrenal axis and transient hypercortisolism.

707. A. Cushing's disease is characterized by hypersecretion of cortisol by the adrenal cortex, while Addison's disease is characterized by hypocortisolism.

708. D. Dexamethasone is used to evaluate the dynamics of the hypothalamic-pituitary-adrenal axis.

709. C. A positive ACTH stimulation test can exclude the diagnosis of Addison's disease and point more toward a pituitary problem.

710. E. In addition, Anti-HBs can be detected by RIA.

711. B. The Australia antigen has been shown to be the surface antigen of the hepatitis B virus, also denoted as HB Ag.

712. B. Hepatitis B is readily spread by HBV (hepatitis B virus) contaminated blood, serum, or secretions on items such as shared instruments used by drug users, hemophiliacs, medical and dental personnel, etc.

713. A. Direct contact with an infected individual, leading to contamination of the hands and mouth, or indirect contact through vectors such as contaminated utensils, is characteristic.

714. A. Anti-HAV, or the antibody to the hepatitis A virus, is present in patients with hepatitis A and occurs in varying concentrations during the course of the illness.

715. B. The RIA method does not provide quantitative data, but rather merely dichotomizes as to whether a sample is HAA positive or negative in comparison with a set of controls.

716. A. T_3 levels are generally low in utero, rising rapidly in the first few hours post parturition. Normal levels are established within several days after birth.

717. B. Reverse T_3 results from monoiodination of the inner ring and plays a role in peripheral thyroid metabolism.

718. A. In order to measure total serum T4 by RIA, extraneous interferences such as binding to the plasma proteins normally present in the blood, must be eliminated. This can be accomplished by acidification, heat, or blocking with agents such as ANS and thiomerosal.

719. B. T_3 is elevated in true hyperthyroid patients as well as those with the entity known as "T_3-toxicosis."

720. A. In primary hypothyroidism, the TSH levels are greatly elevated above normal, whereas in secondary hypothyroidism, due to pituitary insufficiency, the levels will be low or normal.

721. D. TSH levels are usually low or undetectable in hyperthyroid patients and normal patients, and elevated in hypothyroid patients.

722. B. TSH is chemically similar to other glycoproteins such as LH, FSH, and HCG. The production of highly specific antisera has overcome the cross-reactivity problem for the most part, although high concentrations of HCG are still capable of cross-reactivity.

723. B. Monitoring the TSH levels is also useful in the management of thyroid replacement therapy of hypothyroid patients.

724. B. Calcitonin, a calcium-lowering polypeptide hormone, is produced and secreted by the parafollicular, or C-cells, of the thyroid gland.

725. B. MCT, or medullary carcinoma of the thyroid, is a tumor of the calcitonin-producing C-cells of the thyroid and causes elevated circulating levels of calcitonin peripherally.

726. C. Acromegaly, or enlargement of the hands, feet, mandible, and organs, is due to an oversecretion of HGH (human growth hormone).

727. B. The main function of PTH is the regulation of the calcium-ion concentration in the body fluids.

728. B. Hyperparathyroidism can be classified as primary (due to adenoma hyperplasia or carcinoma) or secondary (due to renal failure). Prior to the introduction of PTH by RIA, the causes of hypercalcemia were difficult to distinguish in terms of parathyroidal from nonparathyroidal origin.

729. C. Specimens for PTH determinations should be collected early in the morning (PTH varies diurnally), after an overnight fast, and should be frozen immediately to prevent degradation by serum proteases.

730. D. Prior to the introduction of PTH by RIA, the causes of hypercalcemia were difficult to distinguish as far as parathyroidal vs. nonparathyroidal origins were concerned.

731. A. Gastrin has a wide range of actions in the GI tract, the most important of which is the stimulation of acid secretion by the stomach.

732. B. The patient should have fasted overnight in preparation of a serum gastrin assay. In addition, the blood sample must be separated within 1 hour after collection and the serum stored frozen until assayed.

733. B. Zollinger-Ellison syndrome, or gastrinoma, is characterized by extreme gastric hyperacidity as a result of increased gastric stumulation by elevated levels of gastrin.

734. B. Differentiation of these two disease entities can be made after administration of a gastrin-inhibiting agent such as hydrochloric acid. Gastrin levels in patients with pernicious anemia will fall abruptly, whereas patients with Zollinger-Ellison syndrome will maintain elevated levels.

735. A. Studies have shown that peak serum levels in bile acids occur at 1-2 hours postprandially so that a 90-minute sample would seem optimal. Position does not affect the levels.

736. C. Normal uptake of intestinal bile acids following a meal takes place in the terminal ileum. Damage to this area either by disease, surgery, or radiation may lead to a flat response in postprandial bile acid levels.

737. B. Serum bile acids are elevated in all types of liver disease and cannot discriminate between particular types of liver disease. Once diagnosed, however, the assay of bile acids can serve as a valuable aid in the treatment and follow-up of these patients.

738. D. Intravenous administration is, of course, the most direct route of introducing a drug into the circulation and thus reaches peak concentration the quickest. This is followed by IM and the oral route, which involves interaction with the gastric juice and the mucosal wall.

739. B. This process begins almost immediately after absorption of the drug takes place. In the liver, enzymes act on the drug to destroy its chemical functions, after which it is excreted by the renal route.

740. C. As with all drug levels, there is some overlap between therapeutic and toxic levels and each laboratory must establish its own levels.

741. D. The therapeutic and toxic ranges recommended in the kit inserts are based on values measured 8 hours after the last dose.

742. C. Digoxin is not normally excreted in the feces. Other variables affecting serum digoxin concentrations include hypoxia, acidosis, alkalosis, and serum levels of potassium and magnesium. Certain drugs such as quinidine and verapamil tend to increase serum digoxin concentrations.

743. D. Electrolyte imbalances also can affect the serum digoxin concentrations; therefore, interpretation of the results should be made in the appropriate clinical context.

744. D. Although digitoxin and digoxin are structurally similar, their properties are vastly different. Digitoxin is handled mainly by hepatic onjugation, has a mean half-life of 7.1 days, and is less frequently used than digoxin.

745. C. Serum CK-B levels rise in patients with AMI within 4 to 5 hours after insult, and often return to normal within 24 hours post-insult.

746. D. Serum CK-B levels rise in patients with AMI within 4 to 5 hours after insult, and often return to normal within 24 hours.

747. B. Since CK-B levels are elevated in acute CVA, it is important to exclude patient's brain injury when evaluating CK-B levels for acute myocardial infarction.

748. A. Myoglobin from both cardiac and skeletal muscle is immunochemically identical. Therefore, levels will be elevated in both AMI as well as in genetic or acquired skeletal muscle disorders and interpretation of results should be made in the appropriate clinical context.

749. A. Serum myoglobin levels by RIA will be elevated in more than 90% of patients with clinical and lab evidence of AMI if the serum samples are collected between 0 to 4 hours after symptoms occur.

750. D. Large doses (such as 2 gm daily) of oral axcorbic acid may produce falsely low serum B_{12} levels by radioassay.

751. E. Pernicious anemia and malabsorption syndrome cause low levels of serum B_{12}, while acute renal failure, liver disorders, and polycythemia vera can result in elevated levels.

752. C. Vitamin B_{12} levels are decreased in diseases such as megaloblastic and pernicious anemias.

753. C. Long-term deficiency of vitamin B_{12} can result in megaloblastic anemia, which is a serious disease and if not remedied, can lead to irreversible neuropathy. Pernicious anemia occurs as a result of a deficiency in intrinsic factor and can lead to megaloblastic anemia.

754. D. Intrinsic factor isolated from hog ileal mucosa is a specific reactor substance that is commonly used.

755. C. Since vitamin B_{12} contains cobalt in its structure, radioactive cobalt can easily be substituted.

756. B. Beta lactoglobulin, which is obtained from cow's milk, acts as the specific folate binder upon which the converted folic acid competes.

757. D. All folates are chemically unstable and sensitive to photochemical oxidation. Therefore, special steps must be taken to ensure prevention of oxidation.

758. D. Hemolysis of the sample kept at room temperature for a considerable time sill result in a loss of immunoreactivity of the sample. Patients on insulin therapy develop their own antibodies, and the presence of these antibodies in the serum results in falsely low plasma values.

759. A. The alpha subunit is identical for all four hormones in the same animal species, thus cross-reactivity in RIA procedures cannot be eliminated using the alpha subunit. The beta subunits, however, are hormone specific.

760. B. Lack of increasing levels throughout the pregnancy, or a sudden decrease could be indicative of fetal death, pre-eclampsia, intrauterine growth retardation, rhesus incompatibility, and molar pregnancy.

761. C. RIA makes possible the detection of HCG, a glycoprotein produced by the placental trophoblasts, as early as 9 to 10 days following conception. It is also useful in detecting HCG-producing tumors such as hydatidiform mole.

762. E. Alpha-fetoprotein, a glycoprotein, is a major component of the fetal serum proteins. The normal serum AFP level is less than 15 ng/ml, while in malignant states, levels of 1 μg/ml are not uncommon.

763. C. HCG, or human chorionic gonadotropin, is invariably elevated in nonpregnant patients with trophoblastic disease.

764. C. CEA levels are not elevated in benign breast disease, but may be elevated in benign hepatic diseases such as active alcoholic cirrhosis, chronic and active viral hepatitis, and cryptogenic and biliary cirrhosis.

765. B. An elevated CEA is as common in benign pulmonary disease as in lung cancer; therefore, differentiation by CEA levels is not possible.

766. C. Blood pressure is maintained by the interaction of vasoconstriction and volume factors, all of which are controlled by this axis.

767. G. If blood is drawn from supine patients, the renin levels are likely to be about 50% lower than those measured post ambulation. In addition, a high sodium diet will cause the lower limit of the normal renin range to approach zero, making it extremely difficult to measure, as well as being inaccurate.

768. B. It has been found that the generation of angiotensin I from renin is pH dependent, and several approaches to this have been tried using various pH levels. Incubating the samples at 37°C in the presence of certain agents serves to inhibit the further conversion of angiotensin I into angiotensin II.

769. A. Blood is collected in an EDTA-coated tube so that plasma can be obtained upon centrifugation at room temperature. The sample can be stored frozen until use, but should not merely be placed on ice because inadvertent activation of inactive renin can occur, leading to falsely elevated levels.

770. B. This RIA assay is based upon the principle that the rate of angiotensin formation is directly related to the renin level. The plasma renin is allowed to react under specific conditions with its endogenous substrate to form angiotensin I, which is then quantified by RIA.

771. A. Plasma renin activity measurements are useful in differentiating different types of hypertension and allowing diagnosis of the secondary forms such as renovascular and adrenocortical hypertension.

772. C. Gentamicin is an aminoglycoside or a broad-spectrum antibiotic with a narrow toxic-therapeutic range.

773. B. Measurement of blood volumes, i.e., plasma and red blood cell volumes, is accomplished by radiolabeling of specific plasma proteins and the red blood cells themselves. The antibody-antigen complex is not utilized.

774. D. If the values are accurate (that is, they reflect the *true* value), then the standard deviation of the measurements will reflect the preciseness or exactness with which the assay is capable of measuring.

775. C. The coefficient of variation is calculated by dividing the standard deviation by the mean and multiplying by 100 to arrive at a percentage. A CV of 5-20% in any data set is considered acceptable, and measurements which fall outside of this CV range (more than 20%) should be considered "outliers" and discarded.

776. C. Three control concentrations should be selected to cover the range of reportability of the assay and also to reflect significant cut-off points such as the limits of the normal range.

777. C. A Levey-Jennings chart, also known as a Sheward chart, is a graph which allows a composite graphic visualization of individual control values from which detrimental trends can be detected.

778. D. Although simple inspection of the Levey-Jennings charts may identify shifts in assay performance, statistical and mathematical methods of analysis, such as the choices stated here, are needed.

779. D. Subtle changes in the standard curve shape would likely result from changes in reagent lots, incubation time, or temperature, or other changes in assay biochemistry. Repeated freezing and thawing of standards, such as in a defective freezer, would lead to a uniform deterioration of the curve, most probably causing a downward shift in position, and not necessarily a change in shape.

780. C. The thyroid gland, like all endocrine glands, secretes its products directly into the blood stream.

781. A. Morphogenesis of the thyroid gland is essentially complete at three-month gestation, after which time the characteristic thyroid hormones are synthesized and secreted.

782. B. The thyroid gland is derived from the ventral wall of the primitive pharynx and migrates downward to its normal position between the thyroid cartilage and suprasternal notch. Failure to migrate completely or continued downward migration has been known to occur.

783. D. The isthmus joins the two lobes of the thyroid, while the parathyroids, four in all, are embedded on the posterior surfaces of the thyroidal lobes. The pyramidal lobe is an anomalous variation seen in conditions, i.e., hyperthyroidism.

784. C. Thyroid hormonogenesis requires the concentration of iodide by the thyroid and its incorporation into tyrosine to form MIT and DIT, the precursors of T3 and T4.

785. E. The epithelial cells trap iodide and synthesize hormones, while the hormones are stored in the colloidal portion of the follicle.

786. B. Iodine which is not used is exdreted via the urinary and fecal routes.

787. D. The amino acid tyrosine is extracted from the blood and iodinated to form T3 and T4.

788. D. TSH is secreted by the anterior pituitary.

789. D. T3 and T4 are stored in the thyroid follicles as part of the much larger protein molecule thyroglobulin.

790. E. Triiodothyronine (T3) and thyroxine (T4) are stored in the thyroid until needed. Thyrotropin, or TSH, is secreted by the anterior pituitary and acts on the thyroid.

791. D. When TSH stimulates the thyroid to release thyroid hormones, active proteolytic enzymes release T3 and T4 from thyroglobulin and are then secreted into the circulation.

792. B. T4 is approximately 60 times more abundant than T3 in the bloodstream, but T3 is more potent.

793. A. Although the concentration of T4 in the blood is approximately 60 times that of T3, T3 is several times more potent on a weight basis.

794. B. Lesser amounts are TBPA and albumin bound. Only about 0.05% of T4 and 0.2% of T3 circulate as "free" form, and yet this determines the metabolic effect of the hormones.

795. B. Thyroxine-binding globulin (TBG), thyroxine-binding prealbumin (TBPA), and albumin are the plasma proteins to which T3 and T4 are bound.

796. E. Parafollicular, or C cells, secrete calcitonin, which, along with parathormone, regulates the calcium metabolism of the body.

797. B. This is also known as a negative feedback mechanism.

798. A. Although only a very small percentage of T3 and T4 circulate as free hormone, this is the portion which is metabolically active.

799. B. The anterior pituitary secretes thyroid-stimulating hormone (TSH), which stimulates the thyroid to release its hormones, T3 and T4, into the bloodstream.

800. B. TSH, also known as thyrotropin, is secreted by the anterior pituitary and stimulates the thyroid to release its hormones, T3 and T4, into the blood stream.

801. C. The thyroid hormones T3 and T4 act on bodily metabolism. TSH also increases hormonogenesis by the thyroid.

802. B. TRH, or thyrotropin releasing hormone, is secreted by the hypothalamus.

803. B. The thyroid gland concentrates iodide from the bloodstream, converts it to iodine, and uses it in the synthesis of hormones.

804. A. ^{127}I is the stable form of iodine.

805. B. "Eu" refers to normal; therefore, euthyroid is a normal thyroid. Hyperthyroidism refers to an overactive thyroid, whereas hypothyroidism refers to an underactive thyroid.

806. E. All of these factors are possible causes of hypothyroidism. In addition, metastatic cancer, chronic thyroiditis, iodide excess, and pituitary or hypothalamic injury may cause hypothyroidism.

807. B. The classic myxedematous patient is pale, has puffy face, with fluid retention, and is lethargic. Other signs and symptoms of hypothyroidism are not as easy to recognize.

808. C. The infant born with hypothyroidism, called a cretin, is characterized by lethargy, pot belly, and enlarged tongue. Both mental and physical growth will be retarded if not treated early in life.

809. D. Pretibial myxedema, a pale nonpitting swelling in the tibial areas, and exophthalmopathy is seen in the majority of patients with Graves' disease.

810. C. Primary hypothyroidism, or failure of the thyroid itself, is usually associated with atrophy of the gland or thyroiditis.

811. A. Secondary hypothyroidism, a relatively rare disorder, is usually due to pituitary gland destruction. The thyroid itself is intact.

812. D. Hashimoto's thyroiditis has also been termed lymphoid goiter, struma lymphomatosa, and most recently, autoimmune thyroiditis and is characterized by diffuse lymphocytic infiltration.

813. D. Plummer's disease is characterized by the presence of solitary or multiple autonomous nodules causing hypermetabolism.

814. B. Plummer's disease denotes a hyperthyroid nodular goiter, while Graves' disease denotes a diffuse hyperthyroid goiter.

815. D. A, B, and C are synonyms for the same disease, and exophthalmos occurs in roughly one-third of these patients.

816. A. Both diseases exhibit a hypermetabolic state and decreased levels of TSH, but only Graves' disease produces long-acting thyroid stimulator substance (LATS) in the majority of patients.

817. D. Each of the three methods has advantages and disadvantages, and there is a lack of complete agreement as to the best method.

818. D. Individuals who have a fixation about losing weight are most likely to be patients with thyrotoxicosis factitia. Careful patient history will usually result in differentiation of this from true hyperthyroidism.

819. B. In the hyperfunctioning gland (hyperthyroidism), the percentage localized in the gland is increased, and vice versa.

820. C. The biochemical mechanism by which the thyroid organifies iodine is at present unclear.

821. C. The uptake test provides functional, rather than anatomical, information which would be necessary to detect a cystic lesion. A scan would be more appropriate in this case.

822. B. The radioiodine uptake test has had its greatest success in detecting hyperthyroidism. The test becomes less diagnostic in the low-normal hypothyroid ranges due to regional geographic variations in environmental iodine, which has lowered normal uptake values in the past two decades.

823. B. The iodide will be absorbed through the GI tract more efficiently on an empty stomach.

824. C. The radiation dose from ^{123}I is on the order of one hundred times less than that of ^{131}I. Therefore, in pediatric thyroid uptake studies, it is the preferred radionuclide.

825. B. Radioiodine in capsule or solution form is usually administered orally for uptake purposes.

826. D. Some institutions correct for room background by subtacting this value from the "standard cpm" in the denominator.

827. B. With the increasing use of iodide-containing materials for medicinal as well as dietary purposes, the extrathyroidal iodide pool has become more saturated, thus tending to decrease normal values. Therefore, each nuclear medicine department should establish its own normal range.

828. A. This is a general range. Every lab should establish its own values according to geographic variation.

829. B. This is a general range. Each laboratory should establish its own values according to geographic area.

830. C. Some hyperthyroid patients, such as those with Graves' disease, have such a rapid turnover of iodine that the uptake at 24 hours is less than that seen at earlier times.

831. D. Normal pregnancy, hydatidiform mole, choriocarcinoma, and lithium administration may also cause elevated uptakes.

832. F. Edema and renal failure tend to increase the iodine pool, thus lowering uptake of radioiodine by the thyroid by dilution, whereas iodine deficiency and chronic liver disease (probably with dietary iodine deficiency) will enhance radioiodine uptake.

833. D. Vitamin C has no known effect on thyroid uptake.

834. A. When the extrathyroidal iodine pool is saturated by administration of, for example, radiographic contrasts agents, the administered radiotracer is effectively diluted and percent radioiodine uptake is decreased.

835. D. ^{123}I sodium iodide is the agent of choice over ^{131}I for thyroid imaging due to its more desirable radiation characteristics. Unfortunately, it is, at present, more costly than both ^{131}I and ^{99m}Tc pertechnetate.

836. A. ^{123}I a cyclotron-produced nuclide is unfortunately more costly than both ^{131}I and ^{99m}Tc pertechnetate.

837. E. Radioiodine uptake results at various intervals after radioiodine administration are related to the metabolic activity of the thyroid itself. Pituitary integrity can be assessed by procedures such as the TSH or TRH stimulation tests.

838. D. A thyroid uptake is a numerical, rather than a visual, representation of thyroid function.

839. C. TSH stimulation serves to activate thyroid tissue which may be nonfunctional for extrathyroidal reasons, i.e., pituitary problems.

840. B. In secondary hypothyroidism (pituitary failure), the thyrojd will be stimulated, whereas in primary hypothyroidism (thyroid failure), it will not.

841. D. A patient with hypopituitarism should demonstrate a doubled uptake from the baseline after administration of 5-10 units of TSH for 3 days.

842. D. Normals and patients with pituitary problems will demonstrate an increase in their radioiodine uptakes by a factor of 2 after TSH stimulation.

843. E. Whether the T3 is exogenous or endogenous, the presence of a specified amount in the blood stream will serve to suppress thyroid activity by activating the negative feedback mechanism. Diseases such as hyperthyroidism, which are not under the control of this mechanism, will therefore not be affected and accordingly will not show evidence of suppression.

844. D. Cytomel, or T3, is usually used in thyroid suppression testing, but administration of T4 will yield similar results.

845. D. Failure to suppress by 50% is characteristic of active Graves' disease.

846. D. Cytomel is administered to the patient every 8 hours for 5 days. On day 4, the patient is given a radioiodine uptake dose, which is performed on day 5, usually with a scan.

847. E. The scan will help to elucidate whether a particular hot nodule is under thyroid axis control or whether it is functioning autonomously.

848. C. Typically, the administration of T3 to a patient with active Graves' disease will fail to suppress thyroid activity.

849. E. The TRH stimulation test is really a measure of pituitary responsiveness. If the patient's hypothyroidism is pituitary related, blood TSH levels will not respond to the stimulation, whereas a normal level will rise 6–15 μU/ml above the baseline value at 20–30 minutes.

850. B. In contrast, the TSH response to TRH in hyperthyroid patients is absent.

851. E. The TRH stimulation test gives similar information about thyroid autonomy status and takes only 1 day as opposed to 5 for the T3 study. TRH does, however, have some side effects such as nausea, vomiting, headache, and hypertension, which must be monitored during the procedure.

852. B. Radioiodine which is trapped but not organified within a specified time period will be "washed out" after the administration of potassium perchlorate. Therefore, the baseline uptake will drop accordingly.

853. E. In addition, patients with an inborn error of iodide organification will give positive results.

854. A. In the normal patient, where the organification mechanism is functional, the uptake will remain unchanged or drop slightly. In patients with organification defects such as in Hashimoto's thyroiditis, the drop will be greater than 10% or more.

855. C. Suppression of the baseline uptake value by 50% in patients with borderline high values rules out thyrotoxicosis.

856. D. The TRH stimulation test requires only the measurement of serum TSH levels taken at various intervals after IV administration of TRH.

857. F. The perchlorate washout study and TRH stimulation study can be completed in 1 day, while the thyroid suppression and TSH stimulation tests take several days to complete.

858. D. ^{131}I and ^{123}I used for thyroid uptakes is given to a patient orally in capsular form or solution. ^{99m}Tc pertechnetate, used in thyroid scintigraphy, is administered intravenously.

859. D. ^{125}I, with its 35 keV gamma peak (suboptimal for gamma camera imaging), is generally used as the label in in vitro thyroid tests.

860. D. The thyroid scan gives information about the size, shape, consistency, and position of the gland, as well as qualitatively assessing its functional status.

861. F. The thyroid cartilage and the Adam's apple are synonymous terms, and the thyroid gland is usually located between it and the suprasternal notch.

862. C. The normal thyroid image shows homogenous distribution of the radioactivity throughout the gland. Heterogenicity suggests nodularity.

863. D. When performing either uptakes or scans on the thyroid using $^{99m}TcO_4^-$, 20 minutes is an appropriate waiting period.

864. A. Pertechnetate, in the form of $^{99m}TcO_4^-$, appears to have an ionic radius and charge sufficiently close to Iodide (I^-) that it is handled nearly identically by the thyroid. ^{99m}Tc pertechnetate is not, however, organified.

865. F. The thionamides PTU and methimazole interfere with the organification process, whereas perchlorate and thiocyanate interfere with the iodide-transport mechanism.

866. B. There is no specific patient preparation for scanning with Tc-99m, but previously administered amounts of iodide may block the trapping mechanism, thus affecting the scan. Therefore, a complete clinical history is important.

867. D. Twenty-four hours is the usual waiting period for both thyroid uptakes and scans using radioiodines. A 6-hour interval may, at times, be desirable when using ^{123}I, due to its 13.6-hour physical half-life.

868. D. ^{131}I and ^{99m}Tc, along with ^{123}I, are the most common nuclides used in thyroid imaging. ^{201}Tl has been used in differentiating the etiology of cold nodules seen with radioiodine imaging.

869. A. These goiters occur frequently in older patients, may be substernal in nature, and can be quite large in size.

870. D. If, however, there is evidence of multinodularity, the incidence of malignancy decreases sharply.

871. D. In addition, conditions such as carcinoma (both primary and secondary) and localized nontoxic nodular goiter can cause a "cold" nodule pattern on a thyroid scan.

872. A. Ultrasonography has been used successfully in differentiating solid from cystic nodules, which are possible causes of the nonspecific cold nodule seen on thyroid scintigraphy.

873. D. Approximately 4% of thyroid carcinomas concentrate ^{99m}Tc pertechnetate, which can lead to false diagnosis. On radioiodine scanning, all intrathyroidal carcinomas are cold.

874. C. The 364 keV gamma emission of ^{131}I enables penetration through the sternum for imaging purposes.

875. E. Functioning thyroid tissue has also been visualized in the pelvic area sa struma ovarii, or thyroid tissue within the ovary.

876. E. Both ^{75}Se and ^{67}Ga have been reported for use in Hashimoto's thyroditis.

877. C. Failure of a hot nodule to suppress in activity after administration of 100 μg T3 daily for 7 days is evidence of an autonomously functioning nodule.

878. B. Organification and storage in the thyroid gland are assessed by the radioiodines such as ^{131}I, ^{123}I, and ^{125}I.

879. B. ^{125}I. ^{127}I is the stable form of iodine. ^{123}I and ^{131}I are generally used for in vivo applications.

880. F. The T3 uptake test measures unoccupied binding sites on the thyroid hormone carrier proteins by addition of labeled T3 to serum and measurement of that which is not protein bound. The availability of binding sites is determined both by total amount of TBG, and by amount of endogenous T_4 which occupies some of the sites.

881. C. The majority of the circulating thyroid hormone is bound to the TBG portion of the plasma proteins and therefore is the most widely measured indicator.

882. A. Increased levels of circulating thyroid hormone with constant amounts of TBG will result in more binding sites on the TBG being filled, and less available unbound sites. The T3 uptake and (CPB) T4 tests rely on this principle.

883. B. By increasing the number of available binding sites, less labeled T3 will bind to the resin sponge, thus creating a falsely low value.

884. E. Heparin tends to falsely elevate the T3 uptake results, while pregnancy and oral contraceptives increase the number of available TBG binding sites, thus decreasing the T3 uptake value.

885. F. A decrease in available binding sites, whether the cause be true hyperthyroidism or a decrease due to drugs or patient status, will elevate the result seen on a T3 uptake test.

886. F. The addition of ethanol to serum serves to denature the serum proteins to release T4 and some T3.

887. A. Heparin will decrease serum T4 results while falsely elevating T3 uptake values.

888. B. Any drug or condition which increases the TBG will also increase the T4 value, and vice versa.

889. F. The T3U and serum T4 tests measure available binding sites on the TBG molecule. Alterations in TBG concentration affect these tests accordingly. RIA procedures are not based on this principle.

890. C. Discordant values seen on the T3 uptake and T4 tests due to alterations in the TBG binding capacity tend to cancel out using the free thyroxine index (FT4I), which is simply the product of the T3U value and the T4 value.

891. B. This test is based on the fact that most of thyroid hormone in the plasma is protein bound. 24 hours after administration of radioiodine, the activity in the serum is measured and assumed to be proportional to the amount of radioiodine converted to thyroid hormone.

892. C. This value serves to compensate for interfering substances or conditions which increase or decrease TBG binding sites. For example, when T3 and T4 values are both outside the normal ranges, but in opposite directions, the FTI is normal and the patient is euthyroid.

893. B. The PBI, BEI, and T4 by column tests all measure iodine bound to serum proteins which generally represents serum thyroxine, but may represent inorganic dyes and medications which contain iodine. The T3U test, on the other hand, depends on availability of binding sites on the TBG molecule.

894. E. Toxic nodular goiter, or Plummer's disease, is differentiated from Graves' disease by the absence of LATS. Other autoimmune diseases, such as thyroiditis, will have circulating LATS.

895. D. The entire nervous system is under direction and control of the central nervous system.

896. B. The cerebrum is separated into two cerebral hemispheres by the longitudinal fissure.

897. C. They are the frontal, temporal, parietal, and occipital lobes.

898. A. The major venous sinuses are named the sagittal, transverse, and occipital.

899. E. The confluence is depicted both on the posterior and on the lateral static images of the brain.

900. A. The cerebral lobes were named after the closest overlying bones of the skull.

901. E. CSF provides protection for the brain from surroundings bony structures by bathing the central nervous system.

902. C. There are two lateral, the third and the fourth ventricles in this system.

903. B. There is approximately 40 cc of CSF in the ventricles of an adult.

904. C. CSF drains from the formina of the fourth ventricle into the cisterna magna of the subarachnoid space.

905. B. The internal carotid supplies blood to the cerebral hemispheres: the external to the face, neck, and outer cranium.

906. D. The posterior cerebral artery arises from the vertebral artery, but there is communication between all three at the circle of Willis at the base of the brain.

907. D. The "blood-brain barrier" is both metabolic and anatomic in nature.

908. D. The small intercellular gap between capillaries and surrounding glial cells precludes the usual mechanisms of somatic capillary transport.

909. C. Because of this, detailed posterior images must be accomplished on pediatric brain scintigrams.

910. B. Gliomas comprise about 45% of all brain tumors.

911. C. Even early generations of CT images are far superior to brain scintigraphy in this regard.

912. C. The radionuclide cisternogram is indicated for a CSF leak.

913. C. It takes at least this long for permeability changes in the brain to occur.

914. F. However, ^{99m}Tc DTPA or ^{99m}Tc GHA used in brain scintigraphy may only be administered intravenously.

915. A. Residual stannous chloride may bind the $^{99m}TcO_4$ to the red blood cells causing a blood pool scan. This will lower the amount of unbound $^{99m}TcO_4^-$ available to localize in intracerebral lesions.

916. C. $^{99m}TcO_4^-$ does not enter the brain unless disruption of the blood-brain barrier occurs.

917. D. The dose should be contained in volume of no more than 2 ml and preferably less than 1 ml.

918. B. Preadministration of potassium perchlorate is necessary to block $^{99m}TcO_4^-$ localization in the choroid plexus.

919. C. While limiting the $^{99m}TcO_4^-$ uptake in the thyroid and choroid plexus, the concentration remains high in the salivary glands and thus the activity at the base of the brain images is usually high.

920. B. This will help to secure the cooperation of the patient; ^{99m}Tc DTPA obviates the need to "block" the choroid plexus.

921. A. Imaging should be carried out at least 30 seconds after the appearance of activity.

922. A. The arterial phase is followed by the capillary and venous phases.

923. B. The venous phase then is in effect.

924. A. Unless the patient is suspected of having a lesion occurring elsewhere, the anterior position is routine.

925. B. The camera should begin then or when activity is first seen on the persistence scope.

926. B. A general purpose collimator can be used for the delayed static images.

927. F. Depending on the particular brain pathology in question, the study may appear all three ways even as a combination.

928. D. Meningiomas will cause localized increased perfusion.

929. B. This finding is supported by lack of sinus activity on subsequent static images.

930. D. Of course, there is no possibility of a dynamic study but absorption is quite rapid when made in the flaccid skin between the shoulder blades - the use of a scalp vein is contraindicated because of the possibility of producing artifactual hot spots.

931. C. Conversely, if a gamma camera is properly equipped, a 1500 to 2000 information density image may be obtained.

932. E. A leaded collar is fastened around the patient's neck to decrease body background in this image.

933. B. Obliques or other views may be required to make the affirmative diagnosis.

934. B. This occurs because the blood levels of $^{99m}TcO_4^-$ level off in 30 to 60 minutes after injection.

935. C. The band is densest and widest at the apex of the skull.

936. B. Primary tumors usually occur singly.

937. B. The "doughnut" sign is a lesion with a central void of activity surrounded by a rim of increased activity. It is caused by necrosis in the center of the lesion.

938. A. An asymmetric transverse sinus is a common normal variant with the right transverse sinus predominating more often than the left transverse sinus.

939. E. On longer than usual delayed images, it is not uncommon for the "doughnut" sign to appear.

940. C. With the disadvantages of expensive instrumentation and a nearby cyclotron facility, the clinical impact of these interesting studies remains to be seen.

941. C. While CT provides the best resolved images, radionuclide cisternography provides the best means of following CSF.

942. D. Radionuclide cisternography is used for the evaluation of the hydrodynamics of CSF and the normal and abnormal CSF pathways.

943. E. The 6-hour physical half-life of ^{99m}Tc pharmaceuticals makes it inadequate for delayed imaging.

944. A. After injection, the head is lowered below the hips by using a rolled pillow for 1-2 hours to allow cephalid migration up the spinal canal.

945. B. The dose is limited due the physical characteristics of both these nuclides.

946. B. Commercial or "homemade" flexible plastic tubing sources are shaped to outline the skull and imaged.

947. C. Imaging may be carried out longer if the CSF flow is delayed.

948. A. An extravasated dose will appear quickly in the blood stream and bladder making cisternography impossible.

949. A. Activity should only be visualized in the cerebral convexities and, in younger patients, the cerebral vertex.

950. F. This finding suggests either communicating or normal pressure hydrocephalus.

951. E. They may be removed later for counting in a well counter. A substantial increase in radioactivity over serum levels is indicative of a CSF leak.

952. B. The hepatic artery supplies about 300 ml of blood per minute, while the portal vein supplies about four times this amount.

953. D. Circulating glucose (a monosaccharide) is converted to glycogen (a polysaccharide) in the liver and stored until decreased blood sugar level triggers its release.

954. B. Some reasons for its susceptibility are thought to be due to the spleen's spongelike tissue, proximity to the lower ribs, relative mobility, and its loose capsule.

955. B. Riedel's lobe has been shown to appear in about 4% of patients.

956. C. Hepatomegaly is also a common finding in lymphoma and cirrhosis.

957. A. The Kupffer cells are responsible for clearing foreign particulate matter in the blood stream.

958. B. This function is carried out by the Kupffer cells.

959. A. Splenic hematopoiesis is usually ended at birth, however certain hematologic pathologies may return this function.

960. B. The upper normal limit for the posterior image is 13.0 cm.

961. E. About 50 cc of bile is stored in adults.

962. E. Though providing anatomic information, both techniques primarily provide functional information.

963. B. Both A and C have been used as agents in the past, but due to their relatively long half-lives and energies have been replaced by ^{99m}Tc sulfur colloid.

964. C. This dosage will allow high information density images to be accomplished in a relatively short period of time.

965. E. Factors affecting colloid clearance rates include liver blood flow, the particle size and number, and RES integrity.

966. E. About 10% localizes in the spleen, and about 5% within bone marrow.

967. B. The delay is necessary to allow adequate time for the radiopharmaceutical to clear.

968. B. This larger range is due to preparation factors as heating time, contaminants, and the amount of gelatin used.

969. B. The presence of ^{99m}Tc sulfur colloid in the lungs may also indicate RES activity in the lungs.

970. A. Bone marrow is more efficient at removing smaller particles, while the spleen is better at larger particles.

971. C. Quantifiable blood flow rates cannot be accomplished. However, the relative amounts of hepatic artery or portal vein blood supply to the liver indicates a normal or diseased liver.

972. B. "Cold" areas appear because of space-occupying lesions within the liver or because of decreased function of the phagocytic Kupffer cells.

973. E. This occurs because the majority of the liver's blood flow is derived from the hepatic vein.

974. B. This will allow proper evaluation of portal vein and hepatic artery flow to the liver as well as visualization of any areas of decreased or increased activity.

975. A. Typically, the lead marker has interspaced lead sections of known size to estimate the actual size of the liver. They are commercially available but can easily be made.

976. E. If at all possible, liver scintigraphy should be performed first as the presence of overlying barium will cause false-positive results. A KUB radiograph will determine any barium presence.

977. E. Usually, the inferior portion of the right lobe of the liver is indented by the right kidney only on the posterior view.

978. A. The left lobe is usually anterior to the right lobe.

979. A. The standing position is the simplest way to reduce respiratory motion of the liver and, hence, improve the resolution of the image.

980. E. Prominent skin folds of the obese patient may also cause cold artifacts. Having the patient stand will often eliminate or shift the artifacts.

981. D. Decreased liver function will cause increased uptake of ^{99m}Tc sulfur colloid in the spleen and bone marrow with this disease.

982. C. Typically, the dose to the liver is halved and the dose to the spleen is doubled.

983. A. The shape is usually rectangular with sharp borders. This cold lesion returns to normal usually within months.

984. B. They are usually resolved over a 3-4 month period.

985. C. Hepatomas do not concentrate labeled colloids but reliably take up ^{67}Ga.

986. C. This results in communication between the superior vena cava and the portal vein, causing a high concentration of the colloid at the point of entry and therefore a "hot spot."

987. A. Typically these are from metastatic lesions with breast or colon primary sites.

988. D. Care must be taken to obtain a truly left lateral image when scanning to avoid any superimposition over the liver.

989. A. Primary or metastatic tumors usually cause focal cold areas, but there is little of the colloid "shifting" associated with the other listed pathologies.

990. C. The spleen does not possess polygonal cells and therefore cannot assess function.

991. C. This will typically cause a smaller spleen (7 cm or less) in an adult.

992. E. The spleen is best visualized in its long dimension without overlap of the liver in the posterior position due to the fact that it is a posterior organ.

993. E. The RPO will separate the left lobe of the liver from the spleen; the LPO allows closest camera positioning to the spleen; but the right lateral will cause superimposition of the liver over the spleen.

994. C. The most common cause of functional asplenia is due to sickle cell disease.

995. E. Chronic multiple splenic infarctions will destroy its function and therefore its ability to be visualized with ^{99m}Tc sulfur colloid.

996. C. This is in contrast to the significance of metastatic disease in the liver.

997. C. Sequestration of heat-damaged red cells occurs in the splenic sinusoids and they are not localized by any other organ.

998. B. It is used to evaluate splenectomy candidates.

999. E. Count rates are done at 24 hours and every other day for 2 weeks after radiopharmaceutical administration.

1000. B. Ratios of 2:1 or greater are abnormal, indicating sequestration rates.

1001. C. The kidneys also maintain proper electrolytic balance.

1002. A. ADH—a hormone secreted by neurohypophysis—in part governs renal function.

1003. C. Renal plasma flow is about 700 ml/min.

1004. A. The nephron, the structural and functional unit of the kidney, consists of a renal corpuscle and its attached tubule consisting of proximal, Henle's loop, and distal convoluted portions.

1005. C. The cortex is the outer portion of the kidney containing arteries, veins, convoluted tubules, and glomerular capsules. The inner portion is termed the medulla.

1006. C. The right kidney is usually positioned lower than the left due to displacement by the liver.

1007. F. The three processes are: Water and solutes are first filtered at the glomeruli, then most of the water and some of the solutes are reabsorbed into the blood by the tubules, and finally some substances such as potassium and hydrogen atoms are excreted into the urine.

1008. A. Radionuclides have been used to attempt to calculate plasma clearance values since the 1950s.

1009. D. Several techniques have been used to determine the GFR in both adults and children using ^{99cm}Tc DTPA and computer analysis.

1010. B. Nuclear techniques do not provide the required resolution to adequately evaluate renal artery morphology. This is best accomplished with x-ray arteriography.

1011. D. Ultrasound excels in demonstrating a mass and its internal structure, i.e., solid vs. cystic vs. mixed.

1012. D. $^{99cm}Tc\ O_4^-$ use is restricted to perfusion studies since most of it is filtered then reabsorbed, and interfering bowel background quickly occurs.

1013. A. ^{99cm}Tc DMSA becomes plasma protein bound within the patient and hence is only used for kidney visualization.

1014. D. All of the others are localized by one of the listed mechanisms except ^{131}I Hippuran, which has a combination of tubular secretion and, to a lesser extent, glomerular filtering.

1015. F. ^{67}Ga is an example of A; ^{99cm}Tc GHA is an example of B; and ^{99cm}Tc DMSA is an example of C.

1016. A. A secondary use, though better suited to other radiopharmaceuticals, is to evaluate the patency of the excretory urinary system.

1017. E. This finding contrasts with the use of glomerular filtration agents which do not increase activity with time due to their low tubular retention.

1018. D. This simple step will significantly reduce the radiation dose to the thyroid.

1019. D. The remaining 20% localizes by glomerular filtration.

1020. E. To best study the kinetics of ^{131}I Hippuran, sequential images of 2-3 minutes duration for a total of 20-30 minutes are acquired on a gamma camera's multiformat mode.

1021. E. The thyroid may receive up to 30 rads/mCi of ^{131}I Hippuran depending upon the amount of unbound ^{131}I in the preparation.

1022. F. The three portions are typically expressed in computer-generated graph form from gamma camera data. This methodology has largely replaced the older strip chart/dual or triple probe procedure.

1023. A. Typical computer analysis algorithms of ^{131}I Hippuran studies produce time/activity curves.

1024. A. The activity is primarily in the extrarenal vessels during the vascular phase.

1025. A. This finding is usually accompanied by a decreased GFR.

1026. D. The relatively short physical half life of ^{123}I of 13 hours would result in increased cost especially if kept on hand for daily routine use.

1027. B. The inverse is also true, that is, 140 keV photopeak of ^{99m}Tc will not scatter up into the 360 keV photopeak of ^{131}I.

1028. B. A relatively high 42% of ^{99m}Tc DMSA is in the renal cortex at 6 hours after administration.

1029. B. This accounts for the fact that there is no significant glomerular filtration but rapid tubular cell uptake of ^{99m}Tc DMSA.

1030. B. The gross anatomy of the kidneys and diseases with space-occupying lesions are best evaluated with ^{99m}Tc DMSA.

1031. C. 5 mCi of ^{99m}Tc DMSA is recommended to provide adequate gamma camera static imaging statistics.

1032. E. This amount of time will permit the highest target-to-nontarget ratio.

1033. C. Also, the intensity of the images should be low in order to visualize deep-seated lesions.

1034. C. Renal adenocarcinoma, being a vascular tumor, presents as increased activity on a dynamic study that may persist on static images.

1035. D. Because of its high kidney retention, ^{99m}Tc DMSA is typically administered in 5 mCi or less dosages—an amount which is less than ideal for gamma camera dynamic scintigraphy.

1036. E. The pinhole collimator will obtain magnified images, while the lateral and oblique views help to completely visualize the cortex.

1037. A. Both the cortex concentration and radiation dose of ^{99m}Tc GHA is less than ^{99m}Tc DMSA, therefore the GHA dosage may be increased 2 to 3 times to reach the same cortical concentration of DMSA.

1038. B. ^{99m}Tc DTPA is by far the best and quickest filtered radiopharmaceutical of those listed and is often used for determination of GFR.

1039. C. Because there is little protein binding by this agent, it is quickly excreted and therefore best suited for perfusion and/or GFR determinations.

1040. A. The glomeruli function as semipermeable membranes allowing only small molecular-sized compounds to pass.

1041. D. A relatively high dose is required for adequate imaging statistics, but the radiation dosage is acceptable (especially with frequent voiding) due to ^{99m}Tc DTPA kinetics.

1042. D. The use of a large field of view camera facilitates patient positioning and obviates the use of the field magnifying, but distorting, diverging collimator.

1043. B. This is because of the rapid filtration of ^{99m}Tc DTPA within the renal cortex.

1044. D. Chronic cases of pyelonephritis appear as having a small kidney with markedly decreased activity.

1045. B. More computer images are acquired in order to produce adequate points on a time/activity curve.

1046. E. Any asymmetry of flow on the dynamic image is considered abnormal.

1047. E. Bilateral renal artery stenosis is noted by decreased perfusion in both kidneys.

1048. C. Obstructed systems will not significantly clear the ^{99m}Tc DTPA within 30 minutes.

1049. B. One of the normal findings on qualitative assessments is drainage of activity into the bladder; hence the need of the patient to void prior to lasix.

1050. A. The transplanted kidney is most commonly placed anteriorly in the patient's lower abdomen; hence the patient is placed supine and images are acquired anteriorly for best results.

1051. B. This amount is independent of body weight and is limited by radiation dose considerations.

1052. A. This early first study is used as a baseline for subsequent serial transplant scintigraphy.

1053. E. Although ^{67}Ga and ^{131}I fibrinogen also localize within graft rejections, their physical properties make them less than ideal for camera imaging.

1054. D. These findings are typical in acute transplant rejections although biochemical findings may still be normal.

1055. F. The catheterized methods are direct methods involving instillation of radionuclide or contrast media. The noncatheterized method is an indirect method that takes advantage of a bladder filled with activity from a 2-hour previously accomplished renal scan.

1056. D. Conventional x-ray provides much greater anatomic detail than nuclear scintigraphy.

1057. A. The radiation dose delivered to the patient will be on the order of mRads with the nuclear technique. Radiographic techniques deliver a dose on the order of Rads.

1058. F. This will allow visualization of uretheral reflux during this phase.

1059. D. A high intensity setting is used to visualize a minute amount of reflux into the upper urinary tract.

1060. C. The elimination of bladder catheterization reduces the risk of introducing infection in children with urinary tract disorders. However, A, B, D, and E are advantages of the direct method of cystography.

1061. A. The other major skeletal anatomical division is the appendicular skeleton, which includes the pelvis and the upper and lower extremities.

1062. C. Also included in this group are several of the skull bones.

1063. A. These bones are typically cubic in shape.

1064. B. The periosteum covers all bone except in areas of articulation or ligament or tendon attachment sites.

1065. B. The red marrow derives its color from the red blood cells being produced in these bones.

1066. A. Osteoblasts arise from fibroblasts and, as they mature, are associated with the production of bone.

1067. B. Osteocytes are found in healthy, normal, and stable bones.

1068. E. Most of this calcium plays a structural role in the skeleton.

1069. F. These three form the inorganic mineral hydroxyapatite. [Ca_{10} (PO_4) 6 (OH_2)].

1070. A. The bone scan is relatively independent of changes in calcium homeostasis as the ^{99m}Tc labeled phosphates localize in bone hydroxyapatite crystal structures. This contrasts with a required 30–50% calcium loss before bone x-rays become positive.

1071. B. The ideal bone imaging agent should have rapid soft tissue clearance and low retention to achieve a high target-to-nontarget ratio.

1072. D. A principal gamma energy of over 1.3 Mev makes this radionuclide impractical from an instrumentation and dosimetry standpoint.

1073. C. The technetium labeled phosphate analogs have replaced earlier used calcium analogs (e.g., strontium 85) and hydroxyl group compounds (e.g., fluorine 18).

1074. D. ^{99m}Tc is the least satisfactory agent due to relatively slow blood clearance.

1075. A. Though the precise mechanism is not known, these agents do bind to the hydroxyapatite crystal substructure

1076. D. A, B, and C play a role but the dominant factor is any cause which results in reactive bone formation and increased blood flow.

1077. The organic diphosphonate bonds (P—C—P) are more stable in vivo than the inorganic pyrophosphate bonds (P—O—P).

1078. D. The bladder is considered the critical organ. The dose can be reduced by frequent bladder emptying.

1079. D. Pediatric doses are typically based on weight.

1080. C. The specificity is greatly increased when combined with laboratory and x-ray results and a good patient history.

1081. A. The epiphyseal plates appear as areas of concentrated radioactivity. Uptake decreases as the child ages and bonc growth decreases.

1082. D. One major benefit of the use of ^{99m}Tc MDP over older phosphorus-containing agents is its faster clearance rate and hence faster imaging time after administration.

1083. A. Forcing fluid will help to clear the ^{99m}Tc MDP from the patient's bloodstream and hence lower the background.

1084. D. Hydrating the patient will facilitate clearance from the vascular pool.

1085. A. Few bone whole body images are obtained on rectilinear scanners because of this reason.

1086. C. The tissue attenuation makes anterior viewing the lumbar spine not worthwhile. This region should be imaged posteriorly.

1087. C. A chart or monogram is often supplied by the camera manufacturer to aid in determining proper scan speed.

1088. E. Electronic or collimation masking is used to achieve a rectangular field of view to allow nonoverlapping passes over the body.

1089. B. Osteonecrosis typically presents as areas with no or decreased activity.

1090. B. Other indications include detection and evaluation of bone neoplasms, infection, and trauma.

1091. B. The site can be localized on the patient's skin with the use of a radioactive marker and then outlined in ink as an aid to the surgeons.

1092. B. Multiple myeloma is an aggressive tumor which causes mostly osteolytic activity with little reactive bone formation.

1093. A. The skeleton is especially prone to metastatic spread of prostate, breast, and lung carcinomas.

1094. E. This high percentage is due to the fact that these carcinomas spread primarily via the vertebral venous plexus.

1095. E. These tumors spread through systemic arterial circulation and hence this appearance.

1096. E. Other areas of increased activity noted on bone scans of older patients due to degenerative bone disease are the knees and thoracic and lumbar spine.

1097. D. Certain arthritis conditions can affect symmetrical portions of the body (e.g., both hands or knees).

1098. C. Following trauma, fractured ribs show an orderly uptake pattern along the plane of impact.

1099. B. Some case reports have suggested that fractures become positive as early as 24 hours or, in a small population, as late as one week posttrauma.

1100. E. Pediatric patients require 6-18 months, while elderly patients require varying amounts of longer time.

1101. E. This will distinguish obstruction from patient positioning artifacts.

1102. D. Steroid therapy induces bone mineral depletion and hence the decreased skeletal uptake.

1103. D. The affected bone typically has a 6-15 increase of tracer over normal bone.

1104. D. Decreased or "cold" areas occur due to the avascularity of the bone in these conditions.

1105. A. A combination of ^{99cm}Tc sulfur colloid bone marrow and Tc MDP bone scintigraphy is a sensitive and specific test for bone necrosis.

1106. D. This pattern will occur with widespread metastatic disease or hyperparathyroidism.

1107. F. Breast uptake may be due to malignant or inflammatory disease, lung from metastatic disease from primary bone carcinoma, and brain from CVAs or calcified meningiomas.

1108. D. The sites where these asymmetries are found most often are in the knee joints, shoulder joints, and feet.

1109. A. Therefore all injections should be made at a distance from a suspected pathologic site and should be recorded.

1110. B. The entire extremity becomes diffusely "hot" distal to site of arterial injection.

1111. C. ^{99m}Tc MDP will not localize in bone with osteomyelitis before this time. Gallium scintigraphy is instead recommended.

1112. E. The three phases are examined by a dynamic study followed by an immediate static and 2-hour delayed statics.

1113. A. Cellulitis is characterized by early soft tissue uptake with usual delayed bone uptake, while osteomyelitis has slight initial soft tissue uptake but intense bone activity on delayed images.

1114. B. An activity ratio from the digital image is generated from each SI joint and the central portion of the sacrum. Elevated ratios indicate inflammation.

1115. D. $^{99m}TcO_4^-$ is used for the diagnosis of active synovitis due to hyperemia. Increased periarticular ^{99m}Tc MDP uptake is related to increased perfusion and bone turnover as a result of arthritis.

1116. B. A 24-hour index is used to determine skeletal metabolism by the amount of retention and clearance of the radiopharmaceutical measured by a whole body counter.

1117. A. The lungs also function in ph and temperature regulation.

1118. D. The trachea first divides into the right and left main-stem bronchi and then about a further 20 times to the alveoli.

1119. B. Anatomic knowledge of the individual bronchopulmonary segments is essential for proper interpretation of radionuclide ventilation/perfusion images.

1120. A. Although by no means exlcusive, intercostal muscles and the diaphragm are the principal muscles of respiration.

1121. E. The pulmonary artery originates from the heart's right ventricle, while systemic circulation is from the bronchial arteries which originate from the aorta.

1122. C. There are an estimated 1000 capillaries per alveolus—the functional unit of the lung where the exchange of oxygen and carbon dioxide takes place.

1123. E. An estimated 80-90% of this resistance is in the larger bronchial tubes caused by turbulent air flow.

1124. C. Tidal volume is approximately 500 ml in an adult.

1125. A. Posture-related ventilation changes are due to differences in pleural pressure, different stress, and thoracic support caused by gravity.

1126. D. Commercial preparations of ^{99m}Tc MAA usually have at least 90% of the particles in the 10–40 μm range.

1127. A. Despite this small percentage, caution should be taken with patients with advanced pulmonary hypertension as there is a decrease in the number and patency of aortioles.

1128. B. Below this number, patchy scans may occur; above this number, little is to be gained in technical quality but the chances of toxicity are increased.

1129. B. This is due to the fact that full development of pulmonary arteries and alveoli does not reach adult levels until the 8th year.

1130. A. The average size distribution of these particle preparations are approximately 15–40 μm. The particles are efficiently blocked during their first passage through the lungs as the average size pulmonary precapillary arteriole is 25 ± 10 μm and the alveolar capillary is 8.2 ± 1.5 μm.

1131. C. Some particles do persist in the lungs for up to days where they eventually degrade and primarily are phagocytized by the liver.

1132. D. The microspheres typically have a more uniform size, of 20–30 μm, than the ^{99m}Tc MAA. Both have been shown to produce excellent quality perfusion images.

1133. D. Concerns of radiation dose to the patient of course still exist, but the potential toxicity concerns of these particulates based on number and size outweigh the radiation damage potential with the usual adult dose of ^{99m}Tc MAA.

1134. C. In the upright position, blood flow is 3 to 5 times greater at the bases than at the apex, while a supine patient has more uniform perfusion. Since distribution of MAA is that which exists at time of injection, a supine patient will have more uniform particle distribution.

1135. A. Imaging may begin almost immediately because, except for a negligible fraction, a great majority of particles are trapped with their first transit through the lungs.

1136. C. This would be due to microembolizations of the radiopharmaceutical which lodge in the lung capillary beds, if either nonuniform mixture or blood is drawn back into the syringe containing ^{99m}Tc MAA.

1137. C. Although A, B, and D aid in the diagnosis of PE, they are not as definitive as the nuclear procedure. Arteriography cannot be considered as a screening tool because of its invasiveness.

1138. E. Typically, this often life-threatening disease is caused by small clot fragments breaking loose and then lodging in the capillary bed of the lungs.

1139. E. The chest film serves to identify clinical mimics of PE, while the properly accomplished ventilation study adds increased specificity.

1140. B. Specificity for PE is increased with a chest x-ray to about 85% and to 90% with a chest x-ray and a ventilation study.

1141. F. To aid in the specificity of the diagnosis, ar recent chest x-ray is read simultaneously. A normal x-ray increases the probability of PE.

1142. A. Although an embolus this small is not visualized itself, the affected perfused area distal to the embolus is centimeters in size and is responsible for the lesion seen on the scan.

1143. E. Anticoagulated patients with known PE should have 50% resolution of lesions in about a week, which will be reflected on a repeated perfusion scan. Chronic lung disease will have the same pattern on repeated scans.

1144. A. If the lungs' bases are better visualized, fewer lesions located in the bases will be masked by overlying lung tissue.

1145. E. The anterior obliques are much less helpful in increasing the sensitivity of the procedure and hence are usually not obtained.

1146. A. Both ventilation and perfusion scintigraphy will reflect this overall increase in size finding.

1147. A. Other diseases which may require pulmonary resection are also effectively managed by lung scintigraphy.

1148. C. Because it begins in the bronchus, it has been shown that bronchogenic carcinoma with a small amount of obstruction will cause a 50% decrease in perfusion in that lung's segment.

1149. D. Changing patient positioning from upright to a lateral decubitus will often change the appearance of this "lesion."

1150. C. The patient does not receive an unreasonably high radiation dose as the short biologic life compensates for the relatively long physical life.

1151. F. The first breath image is accomplished for 100K or for long as is possible; the equilibrium images for about 300K; and washout images for 30 seconds/image for a total length of 3-4 minutes.

1152. E. The other listed factors do contribute to the distribution pattern but all play secondary roles to alveolar compliance.

1153. C. ^{81m}Kr's short physical half-life of 13 seconds disallows any washout study.

1154. B. ^{127}Xe has a physical half-life of 36.4 days and principal energies of 172 keV and 203 keV.

1155. D. COPD is the most common chronic lung disease in adults.

1156. C. Fatty livers are prevalent in alcoholics.

1157. E. The ventilation study requires the patient to follow instructions for washin and equilibrium images while attached to a closed ventilation study, thus requiring more cooperation for an adequate ventilation study.

1158. B. Variation in particle sizing will lead to uneven patterns of deposition within the lungs. Better aerosol systems have lessened these difficulties.

1159. E. This will permit noninterference from the ^{99m}Tc MAA as there will be much higher photon flux from the ventilation study than from the residual activity of the perfusion study.

1160. E. ^{133}Xe washout studies are more sensitive for air flow obstructions.

1161. A. Particulate radiopharmaceuticals are trapped in the capillary beds and never reach the left side of the heart and therefore bronchial circulation. $^{99m}TcO_4^-$ offers the best choice for a dynamic study on a gamma camera.

1162. B. This finding may be useful in distinguishing a pneumonic infiltrate from a pulmonary infarct.

1163. B. Although ^{67}Ga is used to evaluate pulmonary tumors, it is also concentrated by other pulmonary disease, making it nonspecific.

1164. A. There are about 100 gastroenteropathies which are manifest by protein loss from the GI tract.

1165. B. ^{51}Cr - albumin is not reabsorbed from the GI tract but is excreted in the feces.

1166. D. Normal patients excrete less than .07% of the dose in this time period.

1167. E. Thus, the occurrence of a sublingual gland is rare, but the probability of malignancy is high.

1168. E. Salivary scintigraphy is primarily a physiologic exam with the anatomic information gained providing little clinical information.

1169. E. The neck is hyperextended with the aid of a pillow to allow as close as possible gamma camera positioning and to best visualize the parotid, submandibular, and sublingual glands.

1170. B. Lack of oral activity after this would be indicative of ductal obstruction.

1171. B. While being sensitive especially for unilateral disease, the appearance of cold or hot lesions is linked to various tumors (primary and metastatic), cysts, and inflammatory processes.

1172. A. Esophogeal reflux may be best determined when the colloid's motility is unencumbered. This is accomplished by mixing with a liquid to be orally administered.

1173. E. If no activity is visualized within 1 hour, delayed imaging may be accomplished.

1174. B. The study may be repeated using radiopharmaceutical administration by nasogastric intubation if GE reflux is also suspected.

1175. A. Food in the stomach will interfere with the motility of the radionuclide.

1176. C. This device is necessary to set a region of interest over the stomach to quantify activity over time.

1177. B. The "tag" is obtained by administering the colloid to a live chicken where it is phagocytized within the chicken liver. The chicken is then sacrificed, the liver removed and cooked, and then fed to the patient.

1178. A. Pancreas imaging is better performed with a CT scanner if available.

1179. A. This low amount is due to the relatively high radiation dose delivered to the patient's liver (25 mrad/μci) and whole body (8 mrad/μci) by the ^{75}Se.

1180. C. This dictates positioning the patient's lower abdomen in the center of the camera's field of view for $^{99m}TcO_4^-$ scintigraphy.

1181. A. Of these only 25-40% are symptomatic. Ectopic gastric mucosa occurs in about 60% of symptomatic Meckel's diverticulum.

1182. B. Positive Meckel's diverticulum should be visualized within 40 minutes.

1183. A. Many false-positives have been reported because of other structures causing a similar appearance.

1184. A. It is administered at the same time as $^{99m}TcO_4^-$ and acts by stimulating secretions of gastric mucosa.

1185. C. The scanning technique used is similar to that for Meckel's diverticulum.

1186. A. All the other modalities do not have as high a yield as the radionuclide study. However, the use of angiography on patients with radionuclide proven bleeding sites is even more specific and definitive.

1187. B. A higher sensitivity for both slow and rapid bleeds has been reported with ^{99m}Tc RBCs than with A, C, or D. E cannot be used for the detection of abdominal bleeds.

1188. D. The intense liver and spleen uptake of ^{99m}Tc S.C. restricts its use to the lower abdomen and GI tract, whereas upper GI bleeds as well as bleeds originating at the hepatic or splenic colon flexure may be detected with ^{99m}Tc red blood cells.

1189. C. Sequential studies may be performed with more injections of sulfur colloid. However, the use of Tc RBCs allows imaging for up to 24 hours after the initial radiopharmaceutical administration.

1190. B. Each time the blood recirculates a fraction of the ^{99m}Tc sulfur colloid will be extravasated while the background is decreasing compared to RES uptake. A contrast of the site will therefore develop over time.

1191. B. This rate compares favorably to that able to be detected by angiography.

1192. A. If a bleed is not identified by then, anterior obliques may be accomplished or the procedure may be carried out for another 15 minutes to allow the transit of activity that may be hidden by the liver or spleen.

1193. E. Different radiopharmaceuticals have different rate constants, e.g., ^{99m}Tc tracers have higher kidney clearance than ^{131}I rose bengal.

1194. C. The pharmokinetics are altered and hence the radiation dose is altered, making the gallbladder and liver the primary targets in patients having obstructive jaundice.

1195. A. This is better evaluated by the use of ^{99m}Tc sulfur colloid liver scintigraphy.

1196. E. Rarely, choledochal cysts may cause biliary obstruction.

1197. D. This will allow adequate imaging statistics without excessive radiation dosage.

1198. A. The gallbladder may remain contracted and therefore will be nonvisualized if the patient has food in his stomach.

1199. A. A delay will usually cause a decrease in the liver's activity due to the transit of the radiopharmaceutical in the gut.

1200. B. The activity progresses through the liver, gallbladder, bile ducts, and finally into the intestines.

1201. B. Nonvisualization implies acute cholecystitis.

1202. B. This will allow enough time to ascertain delayed filling of all structures.

1203. E. This finding may be due to diffusion impedance of the radiopharmaceutical due to viscid bile or sludge in the gallbladder.

1204. A. This same pattern may also occur in patients with a history of alcoholism and/or pancreatitis or in patients on total parenteral nutrition.

1205. C. 100 units of cholecystokinin has replaced the use of fatty meals, which are too inconsistent in terms of their time and degree of gallbladder contraction.

1206. B. The three layers are the epicardium, myocardium, and endocardium.

1207. E. The pericardium is composed of two tissue layers and contains a serous fluid which facilitates heart contractions.

1208. B. Developmental problems of the septum frequently lead to abnormal communication between the right and left ventricles.

1209. E. The right atrium receives systemic circulation and the right ventricle pumps blood initiating pulmonary circulation.

1210. E. The mitral valve is located between the left atrium and left ventricle; the semilumar valves between ventricles and major arteries.

1211. A. The right atrium of the heart receives venous blood while the left atrium receives oxygenated flood from the lungs.

1212. B. The pulmonary artery is the only artery in the body conveying venous blood.

1213. A. The coronary arteries are the first arteries to branch off the aorta.

1214. D. Cardiac output is the volume of blood pumped out by either ventricle per unit time.

1215. A. Approximately 30% of the cardiac output is routed to the liver and gut.

1216. D. The coronary blood flow may be 4-6 times this during exercise.

1217. B. The heartbeat originates in a group of specialized muscle fibers, the SA node, located in the wall of the right atrium. The SA node is also referred to as the pacemaker.

1218. A. The filling phase is called diastole.

1219. D. The ECG has been used as a diagnostic test for approximately 75 years.

1220. C. The R wave being the most obvious wave is used as the "trigger" in an ECG gating device for blood pool studies.

1221. B. The QRS complex represents depolarization and repolarization of the electrical gradient in the left and right ventricles.

1222. D. Chest leads number 4, 5, 6 all lie in the fifth rib interspace.

1223. C. The AVR lead is the only other lead placed on the right of a patient's sternum in a 12-lead electrocardiogram.

1224. C. Occasionally more leads are helpful in difficult arrhythmias.

1225. B. Effective electrode contact is achieved by shaving if necessary and removing outer layer of skin by proper rubbing and washing with alcohol.

1226. A. ^{201}Tl chloride may be used for acute infarcts but usually is not kept on hand for such purposes.

1227. E. All three conditions must be necessary for ^{99m}Tc PYP uptake to occur.

1228. C. Infarcted myocardium does take up all five radiopharmaceuticals, but ^{99m}Tc PYP has the highest ratio as demonstrated by animal models.

1229. E. 15 mCi ^{99m}Tc PYP is also the usual amount used for routine bone scanning.

1230. D. A, B, D, and E may or may not have ^{99m}Tc PYP uptake in the myocardium.

1231. C. Because of this ^{99m}Tc PYP for acute myocardial infarction is most sensitive during this time.

1232. B. Right sided images are not routinely accomplished because of the increased distance between the heart and the camera face.

1233. A. Since ^{201}Tl is cyclotron produced few hospitals have it in stock for acute infarction scanning.

1234. C. An acute infarct will become less positive or even negative at this time, while an old scar will have persistent increased uptake.

1235. C. Increased patient motion because of increased imaging times makes acquiring more counts impractical.

1236. A. Other pathologies appearing as focal hot areas on a ^{99m}Tc PYP scan are myocardial contusions, rib fractures, left ventricular aneurysms, and calcified costal cartilage.

1237. D. Waiting any less could cause problems with background and blood pool activity of the radiopharmaceutical.

1238. A. Blood pool activity may be mistaken for diffuse myocardium uptake at less than 2 hours.

1239. E. Ejection fractions from early beats are high, while late beats show a low ejection fraction; therefore beats in the midportion of the study must be selected.

1240. C. A compact bolus administration followed by a saline flush is crucial for good first-pass studies.

1241. B. Particulate radiopharmaceuticals are not visualized in the left side of the heart, as they are trapped within the capillary beds of the lungs.

1242. D. The relative rapid kidney clearance of ^{99m}Tc DTPA will allow the study to be repeated fairly quickly. ^{99m}Tc sulfur colloid may also be used.

1243. A. Beginning any later may cause a loss of data.

1244. B. Regional left ventricular motion cannot be observed but ejection fraction can be generated.

1245. B. The multicrystal scintillation camera can typically achieve count rates of up to 400,000 cps.

1246. B. Beyond this point overlap of the chambers causes distortion in hemodynamic information.

1247. A. Although the right and left ventricles are superimposed on the RAO projection, they are temporarily separated during the initial transit.

1248. D. Radioactivity enters the right side of the heart at 3-6 seconds and exits via the aorta at 12-15 seconds after injection.

1249. C. Typically, the left ventricle will be visualized within 1 second after the right ventricle in right-to-left shunts.

1250. D. The number of ^{99m}Tc labeled particles escaping to systemic circulation after injection is proportional to the size of the shunt.

1251. A. Left-to-right shunts less than this ratio may not be detected by any quantitative method.

1252. A. Adequate counts for the transmission scan would not be obtained with blood pool activity present.

1253. C. A lesser amount is insensitive for positive diagnosis.

1254. A. The ejection fraction is one of the basic measurements of ventricular function.

1255. E. EF can also be defined by: $\frac{\text{Stroke Volume}}{\text{end diastolic}}$

1256. B. The cardiac output is mathematically defined as CO = Stroke Volume x heart rate/minute.

1257. E. The volume for both ventricles are normally equal and range from 80-100 ml.

1258. E. The normal right ventricular ejection fraction is 40-50%.

1259. A. Failure to increase or to decrease the ejection fraction during graded exercise suggests cardiac pathology.

1260. A. The resulting scan will have overlapped frame data and therefore will be inaccurate.

1261. C. Dyskinesis is a basic type of myocardial focal abnormality detected by first pass studies or equilibrium gated blood pool studies.

1262. D. The RAO position causes overlap of the right ventricle.

1263. D. The gating device acts both as a R wave trigger and as an ECG display.

1264. C. The R wave is an obvious, easily obtained signal that occurs just before (50 msec) end diastole.

1265. A. This collimator provides the best overall sensitivity and resolution without field of view distortions.

1266. B. ^{99m}Tc in vivo tagged red blood cells achieves the best target-to-background ratio, while ^{99m}Tc physical characteristics are ideally suited for the gamma camera.

1267. C. Any less time does not allow the stannous red blood cell complex to form adequately and hence an inadequate red blood cell tag may result.

1268. A. The shortcomings of the in vivo method (not as high a label, slightly less reliable) are compensated for by the extreme ease of use.

1269. D. The in vivo method shows a 75%+ retention.

1270. B. Because of the decreased field of view, the shield's use allows more photons to be accepted from the heart per unit time while decreasing the amount of photons from other areas.

1271. B. A 40–45° LAO best separates the left ventricle from other cardiac chambers.

1272. D. The tilt can be accomplished by using a slant hole collimator or by angulating the camera head.

1273. The ejection fraction may be adequately obtained using a 32 x 32 matrix.

1274. F. The midpoint of the curve representing the least ventricular volume is near end-systole.

1275. B. The amount is limited due to the relatively high radiation dose delivered to the patient.

1276. B. Thallium is known as an analog to potassium because it acts similarly in some respects.

1277. B. They are initial distribution and redistribution.

1278. E. The use of the less abundant (10%) 167 keV photopeak will improve both the sensitivity and spatial resolution of the images.

1279. D. These four views allow adequate imaging of the left ventricle without superimposition by the right ventricle.

1280. B. This system will provide the best spatial resolution and acceptable sensitivity.

1281. D. Limiting the liver counts will improve the target-to-nontarget ratio and therefore increase the technical quality of the image.

1282. E. Without taping, a circular cold "defect" is often present along the left ventricle's anterior wall.

1283. C. With the patient supine and the detector cross table, the inferior wall of the myocardium may be attenuated by the diaphragm.

1284. B. The right ventricle and both atria have much less tissue mass and blood flow than the left ventricle and hence are not visualized in the resting patient.

1285. E. The chamber is not visualized as is the periphery myocardium because not enough tissue is transposed to be visualized.

1286. D. Rest ^{201}Thallium scintigraphy is most sensitive for acute infarctions and sensitivity declines somewhat over time.

1287. B. "Cold" regions on resting ^{201}Thallium scintigraphy cannot distinguish between sites of acute or old infarction sites.

1288. D. Recent improvement in camera resolution and collimation coupled with observer experience has led to this relatively high figure.

1289. C. The test should be as practical as possible without stopping needed medications.

1290. A. This will allow thallium to clear from the blood to reflect regional coronary perfusion.

1291. B. Thallium redistribution occurs in significant amounts 30 minutes after stress and therefore must be imaged within this time frame.

1292. A. Organ concentration of thallium is dependent on perfusion and extraction fraction.

1293. E. The decreased activity is due to apical thinning of the myocardium.

1294. C. These findings are classic, for transient myocardial ischemia is one of the most common reasons for performing thallium scintigraphy.

1295. E. A number of thallium image enhancement and quantification programs exist, though there is little agreement on which is the best program.

1296. E. Precise positioning techniques on systems with the highest resolution and linearity are necessary to produce artifact-free images.

1297. B. While necessarily invasive due to cardiac catheterization, no morbidity or mortality has been reported for early studies accomplished.

1298. C. The technique relies upon data processing and display of blood flow rates expressed in ml/gram-minute.

1299. F. Radiopharmaceuticals for vascular disease are classified as either particulate or nonparticulate.

1300. A. ^{99m}Tc HAM is preferred for the measurement of the relative distribution of perfusion.

1301. E. A typical dose is 0.5 uCi of ^{133}Xe in 0.1 ml of saline.

1302. C. ^{131}I was first labeled to fibrinogen and used in the late 1950s and early 1960s.

1303. F. This nonimaging technique is used as a screening tool for venous thrombi detection.

1304. A. ^{123}I fibrinogen permits whole body imaging, whereas the ^{125}I fibrinogen uptake test is not diagnostic for disease which causes fibrinogen deposition.

1305. A. The lower extremities are marked in 2-inch segments and each counted for 5 to 10 seconds at 1-3, 24, and 48 hours after radiopharmaceutical administration.

1306. E. Heparin may interfere with clot tagging and therefore its use is restricted in venography.

1307. B. Both venography and lung perfusion imaging after are satisfactorily accomplished with this dosage.

1308. D. This aids in driving the radionuclide to the deep venous system.

1309. D. Deep vein occlusions account for collateral formation as much as 95% of the time.

1310. E. This finding is considered a normal variant and stresses the importance of proper tension in the tourniquets.

1311. C. These characteristics allow sequential imaging for up to a week after administration of the dose.

1312. A. A 4.1% mean % administered dose/kg existed for the spleen in this autopsy study.

1313. E. The normal appearance of ^{67}Ga in these areas after obscures the presence of inflammatory lesions.

1314. B. This accounts for the relatively "hot" kidney findings on a 24-hour image on a normal patient.

1315. A. Normal patients have little accumulation of ^{67}Ga at 48 hours but increased within 24 hours due to kidney clearance. This finding at 48 hours may be indicative of hypertension pyelonephritis or interstitial nephritis.

1316. D. A medium energy collimator rated at least to 300 keV is suggested to avoid images with excessive septal penetration.

1317. D. Although the 93 keV peak is the most abundant (40%), it should be eliminated, as excessive scattered photons into this peak will cause loss of contrast and detail.

1318. B. Thymic and splenic activity may also be increased in children.

1319. D. A major drawback of ^{67}Ga is the 6-24 hours wait after administration of the dose before imaging begins.

1320. E. Though relatively high, ^{67}Ga imaging series have shown relatively high false-positive and false-negative rates due to misinterpretation of bowel, spleen, and spine uptake of the radiopharmaceutical.

1321. E. This will present rotation of the upper torso and evaluate the most likely areas of abscess formation.

1322. B. Although the target-to-nontarget ratio improves over time, inflammatory disease will accumulate sufficient ^{67}Ga by 6 hours to allow an accurate diagnosis.

1323. A. These lesions are completely devoid of ^{67}Ga uptake and also appear as "cold" areas on ^{99m}Tc sulfur colloid images.

1324. C. Typically, sarcoidosis appears as larger areas of intense uptake in organs.

1325. C. The difference in the position between the right and left adrenals accounts for slight asymmetric uptake differences of ^{131}I iodocholesterol images.

1326. C. Typical dose administrations of 1-2 mCi of this radiopharmaceutical requires a relatively long time to acquire adequate imaging statistics.

1327. A. A medium-energy collimator-equipped camera must be used to avoid excessive septal penetration of the ^{131}I photons.

1328. E. Lugol's solution does not improve the quality of images but should be used to block free ^{131}I thyroid uptake.

1329. B. The $^{99m}TcO_4^-/^{201}Tl$ parathyroid subtraction technique seems sensitive for detection of hyperplasia, carcinoma, and adenoma but is not specific in differentiating malignant from benign disease. It is replacing older parathyroid imaging techniques.

1330. A. The pinhold collimator allows magnification of these small glands, while the computer enables enhancement and a subtraction study.

1331. C. The usual dose amount for adults is 10-15 mCi.

1332. C. The patient is usually positioned with the partial or full bladder in the field of view which, if filled, could interfere with the visual interpretation.

1333. D. Areas of hyperemia have increased $^{99m}TcO_4^-$ uptake and therefore this appearance occurs with acute epididymitis.

1334. D. The accuracy of testicular scintigraphy in the diagnosis of torsion is about 98%.

1335. C. Testicular inflammatory lesions and vascular tumors will have increased perfusion and therefore increased $^{99m}TcO_4^-$ uptake.

1336. C. The 6-24-hour delay before imaging begins is a distinct disadvantage.

1337. F. Although the technique may vary from laboratory to laboratory, all three steps must be accomplished to properly label the leukocytes.

1338. C. Any focal accumulation of radioactivity outside these areas is considered abnormal.

1339. D. Further localization will continue until 24 hours when accumulation will remain unchanged.

1340. B. Overlying bowel activity is a problem of the use of ^{67}Ga for detection of sepsis but not of ^{111}In labeled leukocytes.

1341. A. The spleen receives a dose of 4-6 times that of the liver and some 35-50% of the administered dose by 2 days after administration.

1342. D. As is the case with most other nuclear procedures, anatomic clarity is better depicted by contrast x-ray studies. The nuclear study better shows lymphatic physiology.

1343. A. The smaller particle size associated with ^{99m}Tc antimony sulfide seems best suited for transport in the lymphatic system.

1344. C. Such an injection allows visualization of the inguinal, iliac, and paraaortic lymph nodes.

1345. B. Too large-sized particles will not be effectively transported through the lymphatic system. ^{99m}Tc antimony colloid is now used because of its reduced size

1346. E. With a proper injection over 70% of the activity should be transported by the lymphatic system.

1347. B. The large blood pool of hemangiomas may be somewhat "sluggish," therefore accounting for the typical normal or negative dynamic study.

1348. C. ^{99m}Tc MAA is also being advocated by some centers.

1349. B. A 20-gauge needle is passed through the abdominal wall into the peritoneal cavity by a physician. Proper needle location is indicated by aspiration of ascitic fluid into the syringe.

1350. D. When both these findings are present, the shunt is considered patent.

1351. A. Suspected areas of malignancies indicated by increased ^{33}P uptake are mapped with the use of narrow, specialized G-M tubes with ratemeters.

1352. A. An aperture as small as possible should be used to aid in the visualization of the lacrimal drainage apparatus (LDA).

1353. A. The patient must be upright as the rationale of the study is that the $^{99m}TcO_4^-$ will follow the path of tears.

1354. B. Any asymmetric findings are indicative of a block in the passage of tears.

1355. E. The destructive beta of ^{131}I actually destroys functioning thyroid tissue.

1356. D. The greatest variance occurs with this biologic component and hence is the most complex.

1357. B. Typical hyperthyroid treatment ranges within 20% of this dose.

1358. A. The fetus definitely concentrates significant amounts of ^{131}I.

1359. C. Too much of the thyroid is destroyed.

1360. B. The complication rate rises above this dose.

1361. A. One of the most radiosensitive organs in the body is the bond marrow.

1362. B. Polycythemia vera is a neoplastic process.

1363. C. Increase in red cell production.

1364. B. An effective treatment will produce a remission that will last 6 months.

1365. C. I. V. injection

1366. C. It is a palliative treatment.